BREEMA

AND

THE NINE PRINCIPLES OF HARMONY

**Also from
Breema Center Publishing:**

Freedom Is in This Moment: 365 Insights for Daily Life

Self-Breema: Exercises for Harmonious Life (second edition)

Every Moment Is Eternal: The Timeless Wisdom of Breema

BREEMA

AND

THE NINE PRINCIPLES OF HARMONY

by Jon Schreiber

Breema Center Publishing
Oakland, California

Breema Center Publishing
6076 Claremont Avenue
Oakland, CA 94618

510-428-0937
Fax 510-428-9235
email: center@breema.com
website: www.breema.com

Photography: George Draper, Berkeley, CA
Bruce A. Barrett, www.brucebarrett.com
Joy Faye Rowan, Hayward, CA

Front cover photograph: Zumwalt Prairie, © Terry Donnelly, www.donnelly-austin.com

Back cover photograph: Bruce A. Barrett, www.earthreflections.com

Printed in Canada

ISBN 978-1-930469-18-1

Library of Congress Control Number: 2006939535

Breema® — Breema is a service mark of the Breema Center.

This book is for educational purposes only and is designed to familiarize the reader with basic principles of Breema. It is sold with the understanding that the publisher and author are not engaged in rendering medical or other professional health service via the book and its contents. The reader must clearly understand that Breema bodywork can be properly learned only in a live setting from a Certified Breema Instructor. In order to become a Breema Practitioner, completion of the Breema Center Certification Program is required.

Real health means one thing —
harmony with Existence.

Discovering the Nine Principles

Throughout many years of teaching Breema, I have always preferred a practical approach in presenting the Nine Principles of Harmony, relying on my experiences of their application in Breema bodywork and in daily life. That also seems the most natural way to introduce them in written format. That's why this book, which includes excerpts from classes at the Breema Center, is not an exposition of the principles in the linear form in which we are generally accustomed to receiving information. Instead, I have tried to create an atmosphere that invites you in, so you can begin to see and experience the Nine Principles for yourself.

The principles are introduced here as integral elements of Breema's comprehensive philosophy of life. They cannot be grasped all at once. They reveal themselves to us gradually, as our interest and desire grow stronger. Through your own experiences you can *taste* the principles, one by one, and all at once, in a moment of being present. The more of these moments you have, the more your understanding of the principles grows.

The principles themselves are actually formless. Their observable, describable aspects are only hints of their essential quality, which is Timeless, and realizable in the moment. Each principle is itself, and, at the same time, all nine. Though we refer to them with words, their meaning is not in the words we use to delineate them. It's in the atmosphere of Existence they connect you to, in the *taste* of Existence you discover within yourself. When you have new insight into a principle, you'll find that it comes first as a *taste*, prior to any verbal description.

The principles are like a map that enables you to discern the all-encompassing unifying principle of Existence, the Law of Unity. But don't become fascinated with the map. Get in your car and drive! The principles are for you to use, to apply, whenever and wherever you can. That's how they can help take you where you want to go. And when you arrive, you find yourself.

Jon Schreiber

Always and everywhere,
it is possible to taste
our own existence.

As one of the members of the core group that worked with Jon Schreiber to establish the Breema Center, I am happy that this book has come to your hand. If, as a result of reading it, you become interested enough to find a Breema practitioner and experience Breema, or to take a Self-Breema or Breema class, you are on your way to discovering a new and magical relationship to life.

The bodywork and exercises that I contributed to the group many years ago have maintained their original purity and vibrancy. Thanks to the dynamic work of the Breema Center, they now fulfill an essential purpose that exceeds yet enhances their initial use as catalysts for physical and psychological balance and vitality.

Self-Breema exercises, Breema bodywork, and the Nine Principles of Harmony have become the cornerstones of a direct and practical system for introducing people to the art of being present and the transformational teaching of unity which we call Breema—

Being, **R**ight now, **E**verywhere, **E**very moment, **M**yself, **A**ctually.

Breema is universal and has great potential value to anyone with a sincere interest in Truth, because it's a practical road to Self-understanding. Breema's timeless principles are applicable to every situation in life, and they open us to the possibility of awakening to the essential unity of Existence in this very moment.

The Breema Center is the hearth, the source that maintains, nurtures, and expresses the deepest and most comprehensive understanding of Breema, Self-Breema, and the Nine Principles of Harmony. That's why, like other dedicated instructors, I never forget that I am still a student.

Malouchek Mooshan

*Breema is a teaching of the heart,
an expression of the unifying principle
of Existence.*

*Its purpose is to create harmony and balance
between your mind, feelings, and body,
and in your relationship to yourself,
to others, and to all life.*

Preface

Only a fraction of the real essence of Breema can be communicated to the mind. Breema speaks much more effectively to your body. Through receiving Breema bodywork, or by practicing Self-Breema exercises or the bodywork sequences in a class, you begin to see what this is all about. You begin to experience Breema's philosophy and principles in your body. This direct experience bypasses your mind and feelings, and helps them become open and receptive, because you've already had a taste of what Breema truly is.

Receptivity is a universal currency. When you have it, higher dimensions of knowledge become available to you, and your Being is nurtured. Then this book, which includes material excerpted from Breema classes over the years, can really talk to you. Breema speaks the language of your Being. You hear it from inside yourself, as though you are expressing a hidden understanding that has always been a part of you. That expression harmonizes your mind, feelings, and body. Then you can see that Breema is totally practical. Its entire philosophy can be verified.

Although you can get a lot out of this book, I must tell you in all honesty that the words printed here are containers. To open them up and extract their meaning, you need to experience Breema bodywork for yourself. The bodywork offers some of the essential support you need to bring this understanding directly into your life.

If it were possible to teach the bodywork, even in a limited fashion, in a book, I would happily do so. But to learn Breema, the direct presence and atmosphere of an instructor who has for years practiced the bodywork and worked with the philosophy and the Nine Principles is indispensable. Without that, the movements and sequences are merely empty form, devoid of their inner content.

Be nurtured by this book. Use it and take a step. When you are ready for more, find a Certified Breema Instructor and receive a session or take a class. That's how you start to really learn the language of Breema, which is actually your own native tongue.

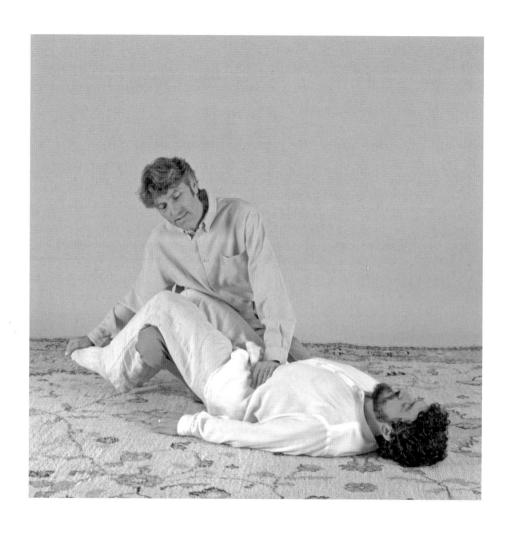

Introduction

Breema slowly unfolds and deepens as one practices it. Breema and Self-Breema exercises express the Nine Principles of Harmony upon which they are based. These principles are distilled from a profound understanding of the universal laws that govern life, and consequently, the body, its health, and its relationship to the energetic and physical aspects of the universe. The philosophy of Breema is derived from these same laws. While, in its scope, it takes into consideration the four levels of Existence: matter, energy, Consciousness, and Awareness, and their interrelationships and essential unity, Breema is ultimately practical, and asks its students to take nothing on faith, but to accept as truth only that which they are able to verify for themselves.

Breema is a truly hologenic system—each principle contains all the other principles within it. Every movement of each bodywork sequence simultaneously calls for the application of all the principles, so by practicing any sequence, one can eventually discover every principle. This process of deepening our understanding is endless, and eventually can provide a definite direction for our lives, as we take a step toward Self-understanding. When we unify body, mind, and feelings, we have the possibility to realize our essential nature. We make understanding our own by living it.

The meaning of Breema is hidden from you, even when it's written and laid out in front of you to read. But as you apply it in your life, the meaning reveals itself. It's like an acorn. You can't see that it contains an oak tree. But if you give it the right conditions, put it in the soil and water it, the mighty oak tree eventually shows itself. The Nine Principles are seeds. You have to give them conditions in which they can sprout. You have to live your life with them, apply them in your life. Then their meaning reveals itself to you. Take them into your life and they become part of you.

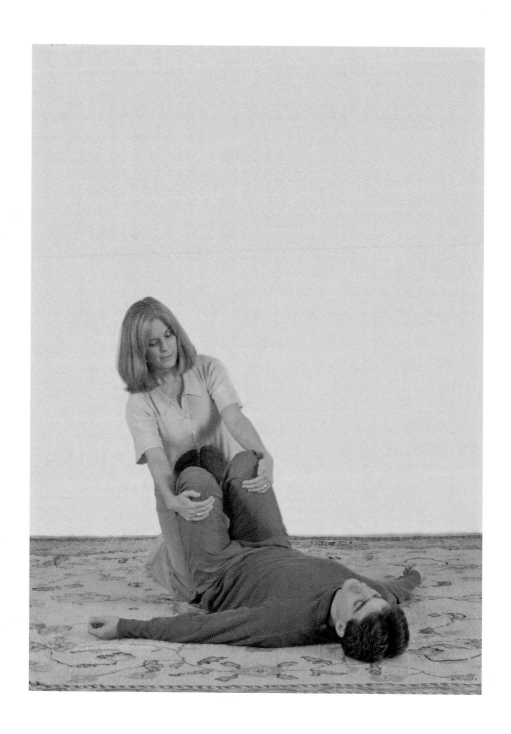

The Nine Principles of Harmony

BODY COMFORTABLE

When we look at the body, not as something separate, but
as an aspect of a unified whole, there is no place for discomfort.

NO EXTRA

To express our True nature, nothing extra is needed.

FIRMNESS AND GENTLENESS

Real firmness is always gentle. Real gentleness is always firm. When we are
present, we naturally manifest firmness and gentleness simultaneously.

FULL PARTICIPATION

The most natural way of moving and living is with full participation. Full participation
is possible when body, mind, and feelings are united in a common aim.

MUTUAL SUPPORT

The more our Being participates, the more we are able to support life and recognize
that Existence supports us. Giving and receiving support take place simultaneously.

NO JUDGMENT

The atmosphere of nonjudgment gives us a taste of acceptance of ourselves
as we are in the moment. When we come to the present, we are free from judgment.

SINGLE MOMENT/SINGLE ACTIVITY

Each moment is new, fresh, totally alive.
Each moment is an expression of our True nature, complete by itself.

NO HURRY/NO PAUSE

In the natural rhythm of life energy, there is no hurry and no pause.

NO FORCE

When we let go of assumptions of separation, we let go of force.

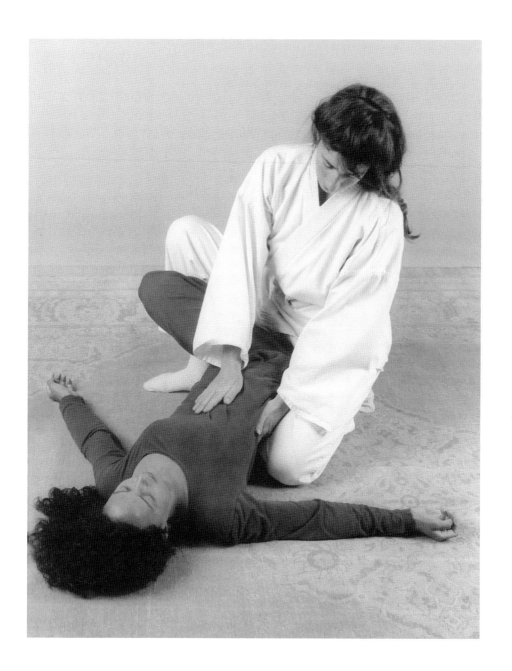

The Nine Principles of Harmony make Breema bodywork unique. They distinguish it from all other methods, even those which include movements that appear to be similar. Yet, the principles of Breema are universal. They can be applied to other techniques and methods of bodywork, health improvement, health maintenance and, in fact, to any activity in life. They can be useful for everyone, not just for those who have an interest in bodywork. You can begin, in your own way, to apply those principles with which you find an inner resonance. If you find the principles inspiring, you will eventually want to support your study by participating in a class or workshop, because both practicing and receiving Breema bodywork are extremely helpful for deepening your Self-understanding.

The first principle of Breema is Body Comfortable. This process starts even before you touch the recipient's body. Take a few breaths, and experience that your body is breathing, and that your body has weight on the ground. Almost immediately you can experience the refreshment of becoming available to yourself and to your immediate situation. Now, you're ready to touch your partner.

Many sequences begin with holding the instep/heel area of your partner's feet. According to principle, you simply place your hands where they feel most comfortable to you. Your hands make complete contact as they gently mold to find a perfect fit with the contours of your partner's feet, without any tension. The practitioner constantly allows their own body to find a position of comfort and support, without compromise. Breema sequences are exactly suited to an experience of comfort for both practitioner and recipient.

Although simple, the principle of Body Comfortable is dynamic. By continually returning to your own body's comfort and the registration of your own weight and breathing, several beneficial things happen. Your energy is renewed and refreshed. As you practice, your body lets go of tension. You're allowing yourself the opportunity to fully partici-

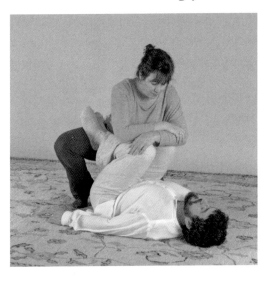

pate in what you're doing. By focusing on the comfort of your own body, you're giving the recipient what their body needs, too. Breema doesn't use force. Your body leans in using only its natural weight, while at the same time supporting and stabilizing the recipient's body. Both bodies receive the security they need to release tension and to experience their natural state of vitality.

The principle of Full Participation is a natural correlate of Body Comfortable. The practitioner's every movement is made with the whole body, with "every single cell of the body participating." Some sequences require raising and rotating both of the recipient's legs or bringing the recipient from a supine to a sitting position. You can accomplish even these seemingly difficult movements without any tension or strain by using your whole body, instead of relying on the isolated muscular efforts of your arms or hands. All of its movements are made effortless, because **Breema doesn't ask the body to do anything that is not natural for it.** The body loves to do Breema movements, because you let your body stay comfortable and move with the whole body.

The *knowing* that *I have a body* becomes the practitioner's center of balance and vitality. When you have this knowledge, you can do Breema simply, with the joy of full participation in your body's activity. Connection to the knowledge that *there is a body* is simple and natural, without any "extra." It is not achieved through concentration, but by returning to the experience of your body's weight, breathing, and comfort.

When you receive Breema, or if you watch someone doing the body-work, you can experience and also see that the practitioner's hands are relaxed and free of tension, yet they touch without hesitation and always make full contact with the recipient. This is *the Breema touch,* which results from the principle of Firmness and Gentleness. Firmness comes from the registration of the relaxed weight of the body, while gentleness comes from the practitioner's presence and availability.

The cornerstone principle of Breema is No Judgment. Rather than focusing on the recipient, the emphasis is always on the experience of your own body. This nonjudgmental approach includes the practitioner as well as the recipient, as both are supported to benefit from an atmosphere of acceptance. This principle says: "Don't try to fix anything. Don't fight sickness—increase vitality!" There is no need to impress others, and consequently no need for worry, anxiety, or criticism. When you do Breema, you're doing it for yourself. Nothing "extra" is needed. You can simply be alive and present. The atmosphere that is naturally created nurtures both giver and recipient, allowing them both to let go of tension and become vital and relaxed.

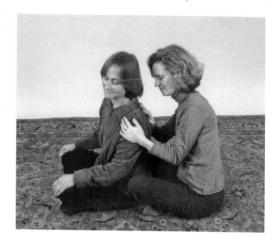

The Breema principles, applied in daily life, can make us free of the *conceptual* body—the ideas and images of our body that we carry in our mind. The conceptual body is divided into many parts—hands, arms, liver, legs, etc. We "see" these separate parts as though they are distinct entities. We label them and identify with them. We forget they are part of a whole system. Breema encourages you to relate naturally to your physiological body (the body that you carry through life) as a dynamic matter-energy combination. You become less and less subject to the ideas you've acquired about the body, and instead, rely on your experience of your body.

In the same way, you are guided to discover the natural function of the mind—to receptively register the body's manifestations. This naturally functioning mind is very different from the mind we are accustomed to. The natural mind is receptive and available, and functions cooperatively with the body.

After your body and mind are balanced, it becomes possible for the feelings to function in their natural state. Instead of swinging between pleasant and unpleasant states, the feelings learn to be calm and balanced, lending a sense of supportive presence to the unified activity of the mind and body.

As a result, we function with our mind, body, and feelings in harmony, and we experience the unity of our three aspects. This unity serves as a foundation for the development of a unified Consciousness which can see things as they are.

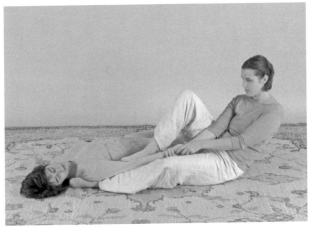

Ultimately, Breema is much more than a method. It is a natural, joyful, and harmonious response to Existence.

Work with one of the Nine Principles,
again and again and again,
and you may get a taste.
That means the inner atmosphere
of that principle is also in you.

*We are "asleep" because
we believe we exist independently
of the unity of Existence.*

*To **wake up** means to know Existence
exists as one unified whole.*

Breema is about self-knowledge, self-understanding, self-actualization, and self-transformation. What does bodywork have to do with it? Why do we receive Breema bodywork, and practice Breema and Self-Breema? Because we are not equipped to receive the truth through our mind or feelings.

We rely on our mind and feelings, but they don't have the capabilities we imagine they do. We are already filled up with fragmented and incorrect knowledge, which we have acquired in a disorganized and haphazard way. This makes our mind and feelings chaotic. In other words, we have been conditioned. We are crystallized. This can't be neutralized by another thought, another philosophy, because we automatically restructure it to fit our conditioning. We can't help it. We've been conditioned to mechanically perpetuate our crystallized ways of thinking and feeling.

How do we become free of our conditioning? Through the process of decrystallization. Unless our body starts to become decrystallized, our mind and feelings never will. We receive Breema bodywork to give our body a chance to have a new experience it's never had before. Because every touch in Breema is based on the Nine Principles of Harmony, it's a brand new experience that can't be mechanically processed by our conditioned reactions to sensory input.

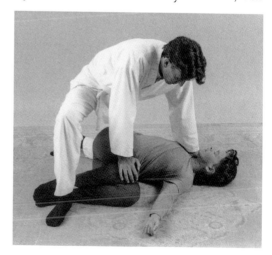

We practice Breema bodywork and Self-Breema to digest what we've heard and read about the philosophy of Breema, so it won't just stay in our mind and feelings. We digest it by putting it into practice. We practice Breema to *experience* Body Comfortable, to *experience* Single Moment/Single Activity. We wish to *taste* the *existence* of the body. We wish to taste an Inner Authority that's free from our mind, our emotions, and our sensations. We want to receive a *direct* impression of reality, without going through the filters of our mind and emotions.

Giving and receiving Breema is an opportunity to let go of our conditioning. The experience of Breema in our body lessens our unconscious identification with our crystallized "knowledge," while depositing in us a hologenic and organized knowledge that is the imprint of the taste of the Nine Principles on us.

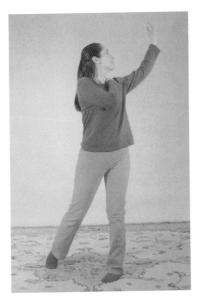

The more we experience it, the more we become capable of receiving life energy consciously, instead of only mechanically.

We've been conditioned to never be present. We're always in the past or future. So we don't know we exist, and we receive life energy mechanically, without knowing it. We work with the Nine Principles in order to taste our existence, in order to have *new* thoughts, *new* feelings, and a *new* posture towards life.

When you receive a Breema session, wordlessly you receive this message—you are not what you *think* you are. And you get a taste of what you *are*. In that short taste of freedom from your conditioning, you are filled up with life energy that lights you up from the inside.

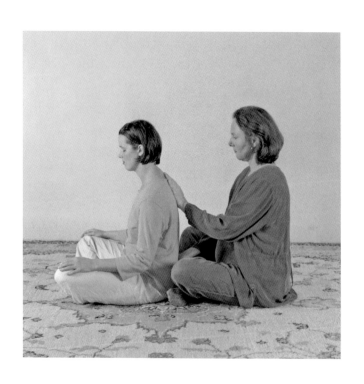

When my mind, feelings, and body
function together as one unit,
I have my own center.

We do Breema bodywork to practice the Nine Principles. While you are practicing, you have a chance to receive a nonverbal taste. You can receive a taste *before* the mind tries to tell you "this is it," before it translates that taste into words. You discover that there is another way besides thought to relate to life.

At first, we are so conditioned, our mind is so conditioned, it blocks us from receiving any glimpse of reality. Breema makes it possible for you to discover a dimension of yourself that you are not familiar with. When your mind, feelings, and body are all present and working together, Conscious energy is present. You experience it as a taste. If you experience taste often enough, you can readily recognize that presence, and the atmosphere it creates. Then it becomes possible to have a taste when you're walking down the street, when you're engaged in any activity. But if you take Breema as just bodywork, without applying the Nine Principles, it doesn't give you that. Bodywork doesn't produce taste. You have to make it a practice of applying the Nine Principles. And once you know what taste is, Breema continues to help you by increasing your receptivity to Conscious energy.

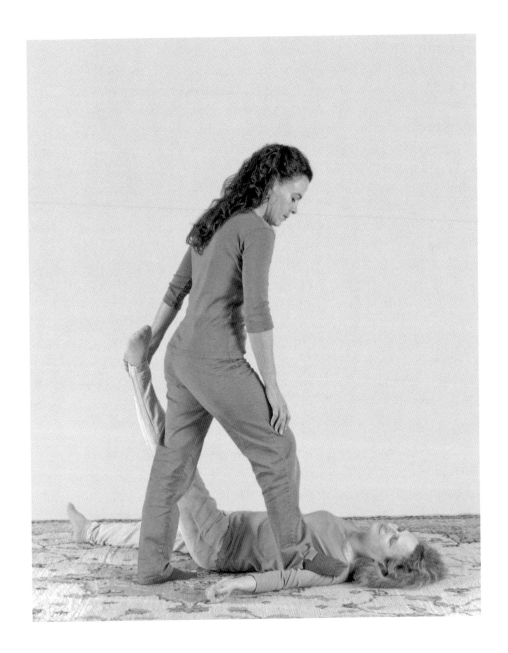

Each of the Nine Principles has many dimensions. If you apply a principle in the dimension you are in, it leads you to another dimension, finer than the previous one. This is why the principles are directional. You can start wherever you are. Take the principle of Body Comfortable, for example. Let's say you are a bit tense. You do something to make your body a little more relaxed. That's a step towards Body Comfortable. But it's not the whole thing, because the body is not what we see with our eyes. It's not what we think it is. The reality of the body is just vibration, just light. The body has many dimensions, and so does the principle. Even when you make what you're used to considering your "physical body" comfortable, your mind may still have a lot of unpleasant thoughts. You can't really call your body comfortable with that type of mind. So you continue to work with the principle and quiet your mind a bit. But there may still be turmoil in your feelings. So you can't really say you have Body Comfortable. You have to do something to balance your feelings, too. You have to breathe, come to the body, and stay with it until your mind is quiet, feelings are calm, and you become present. You can call that Body Comfortable. But still, there are many dimensions above that. You never reach a level from which you can't still take another step.

Every principle has this directional quality. Look at Full Participation. Say I'm shaking hands with someone. I let my hand become more comfortable, so it makes more contact with the other person's hand. That's participating more fully. Now I let the weight of my body come to my arm and hand. That's another step, and if that's as far as I take it this time, that should be accepted as Full Participation. But there is a lot further I could go. I could see that my mind is elsewhere. So I bring it to the activity of my body. That's even more Full Participation. I keep going until I come to the dimension of Consciousness. Consciousness also has to participate for it to really be Full Participation. I have to have a taste of my own existence. Because that is Consciousness. What we usually call consciousness is just mechanical consciousness, not really Consciousness, because the knowledge that *I exist* is lacking. Only when I am conscious of the fact that *I exist* and I'm tasting it, can I really say I am Conscious. If that Consciousness is present when I'm shaking hands, I am fully participating.

Still, it's not total. The dimension of Awareness has to enter. In Awareness, we enter into Unity. Not only am I conscious of my own existence, I see my existence is a part of a greater total Existence that includes everything. This really makes it Full Participation.

But each step, from the moment I remember, can be accepted as Full Participation. Wherever I am, I can always take one step towards what I wish to be.

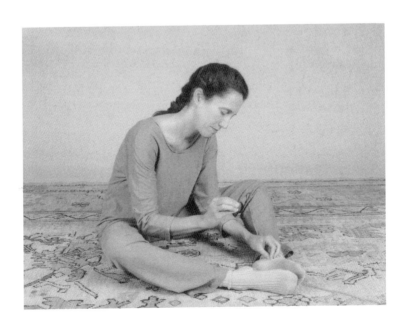

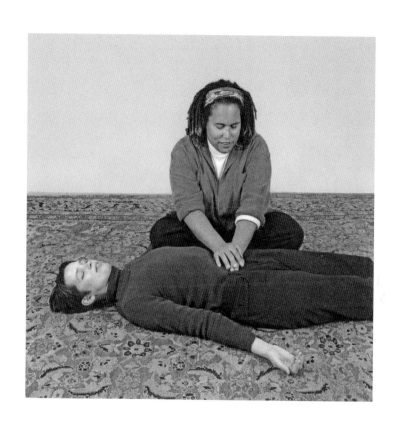

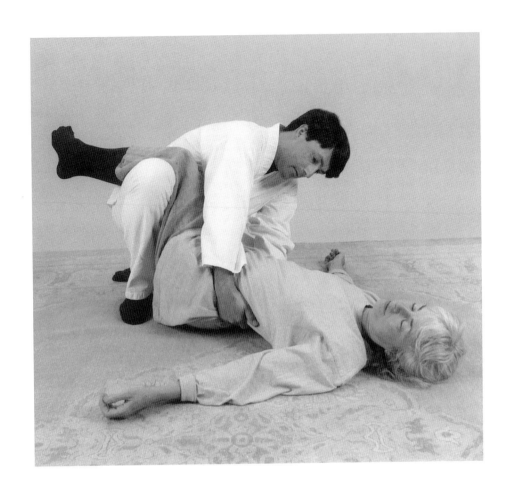

To do Breema, you need to be ordinary. The magic of anything is the fact it exists. If you're looking for magic, you'll find it in the knowledge that you exist. Breema is a universal principle. It doesn't belong to anyone in particular. All that is needed is sincerity, honesty, and simplicity.

When I am alive,
When I am alert,
When I am connected to the commonsense and
instinctive wisdom of my body,
Whatever I do is Breema.

You don't have to force your body to be comfortable. In fact, Body Comfortable means accepting the condition of the body as it is. Through acceptance of the body and its condition, you may discover that you are not this body.

It's very simple to start working with Body Comfortable. By letting go of a tiny bit of tension, you are making your body a little more comfortable. You're going in the right direction.

But your feelings are in turmoil. So you can't say you have Body Comfortable. You have unnecessary thoughts in your mind. Is that Body Comfortable? It isn't. The more you look, the more you see that the principle is endless. To be truly comfortable means to be what you are in reality, unified with the Totality.

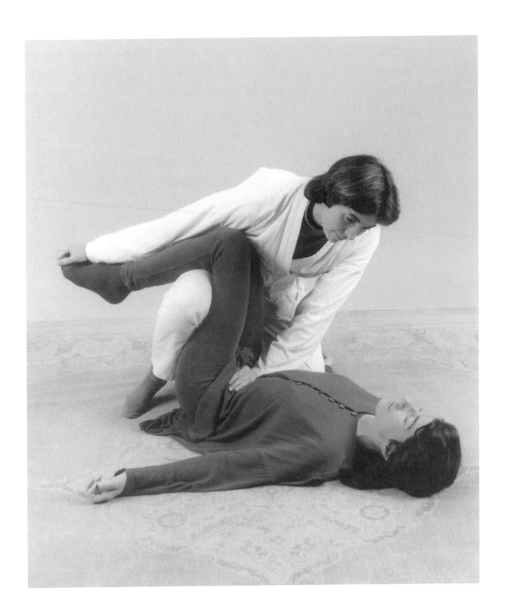

The first thing we need in order to work with No Judgment is to see that we judge everything all the time, without exception. Our mind automatically comments on everything we see. It associates every single thing with something else. We live inside this associative mind, so we don't connect to the reality of things.

Seeing that we're always judgmental isn't enough, though. We have to see it so clearly that there's no doubt left that it is so. Then we can *accept* it. The more we can see and accept it, the more chance we have to discover something in us that can be nonjudgmental. That part of us doesn't judge, it understands.

To be nonjudgmental, drop comparison.
Then there is acceptance, and receptivity
to a higher dimension of consciousness.

The body is a living, dynamic phenomenon
that is constantly changing—
an energy system connected
to all levels of Existence.

The definite knowing that *I have a body* is not dependent on tension, physical sensation, or physical location. At first, these may be part of our experience. As our experience increases, it becomes freer and freer, until only the knowledge of *there is a body* remains. This knowing doesn't have a sense of separation, a line separating "me" from that which is "outside of me." In fact, we are more connected to our surroundings. The knowledge of *I have a body* is the beginning of the knowledge that Existence exists.

When we have the definite taste of *I have a body* or *there is a body*, there is no longer any need to emphasize one part of the body over any other part. That taste is a *knowledge* which is equally the property of every cell of the body. Every cell of the body is working together, and the *knowledge* of this unity is your consciousness. When you are connected to this knowledge, the energy you use to do any activity is continually replenished.

Only when the knowledge of *there is a body* is present in us, is it possible to have new, uncrystallized postures and movements. These uncrystallized physical manifestations act to decrystallize our mind and feelings, so we can have new thoughts and feelings. When body, mind and feelings are experienced simultaneously, we have a sense of *presence*. The mind is receptive and clear. The feelings are centered and free. The body has original, organic sensations, and flexibility. These qualities should not be

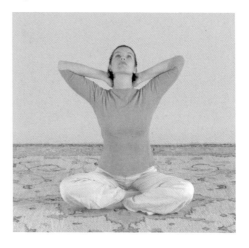

searched for or imagined. When they become present, they let us know. That knowing eventually becomes *Being-knowledge*. This harmonizing knowledge is the threshold that leads to freedom from what we think we are, and moves us toward what we actually are, toward the knowledge of *I exist*. Although *I exist* has a particular taste, it excludes nothing and is a part of Existence as a

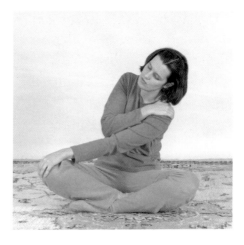

whole. It is the beginning of the profound understanding of the unity of all things that all religions and true science have as their aim.

It is important to rely on your own experience, with full acceptance, no matter how small your experience is. Receive it as a precious gift given by Existence to help you become a unified presence, belonging to the whole. Let your small experiences remain treasures, gifts given to

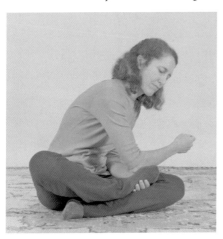

you. It isn't really necessary to talk about these experiences, because no matter how small they are, they announce themselves through their own emanation and radiation. Just enjoy being ordinary, and be grateful you're on the right track.

The energy gained from these small moments can be used in your ordinary life to accomplish some of the things you've wished to do, things that have been put off through inertia and the tendency to postpone "for later." In due time, these small accomplishments make us capable of bigger accomplishments, like losing our false sense of specialness and importance, and gaining an accurate posture of respect for oneself as a *Being-participant* on the Earth.

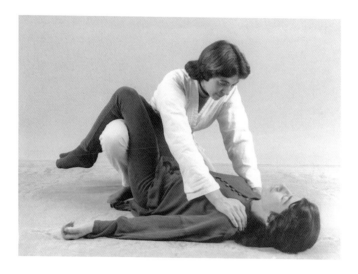

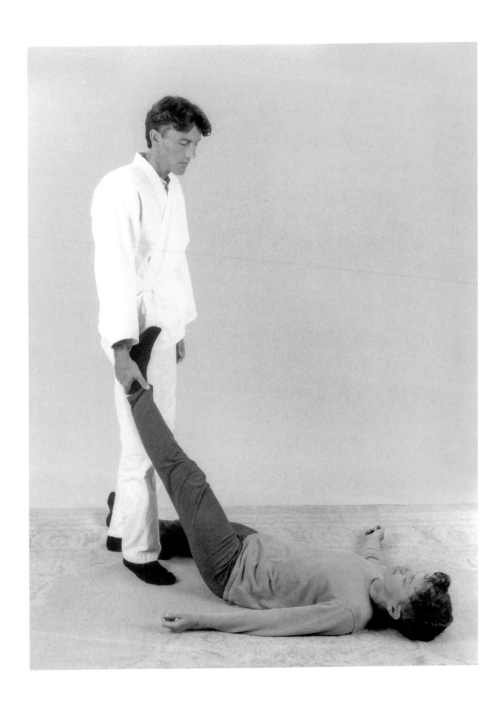

Once you register the fact *there is a body,* you will see that most of the time you are not connected to this knowledge. When you see that, you have to be grateful, because that knowledge is your aim. Seeing you don't have it means you can take the next step. Maybe that step is to experience the weight of your body, or to know you are breathing. At any given moment, your *aim* is something you can do, not something impossible. That way, you can always take a step in the right direction.

When we say Earth, we're not talking philosophically about the planet. We're talking about *our* Earth—our own body. When we're connected to the knowledge of *there is a body,* we are on the Earth.

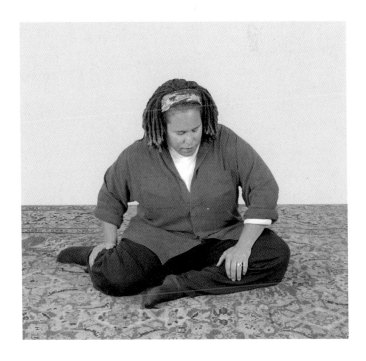

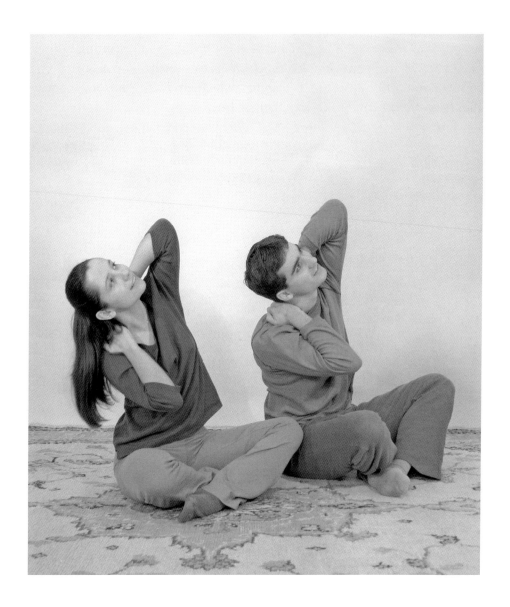

Moment and Breema are two words with the same meaning. When your aim is to be present while your body is active, you are doing Breema. You only need to wish to be present, and express your wish by taking a step in that direction. That's Breema.

Why is being present so important? Because to get the best out of anything in life, you have to give your best. And that is only possible when you are present. To be present means to know you *exist*.

When you drop the past and future, you drop extra. Extra is everything that's not needed in this moment. Then, there is a presence in the present. You can call that presence self, or reality, or God. And you belong to it. You are part of it.

Breema means connection to that. It's not dependent on the bodywork, but at the same time, the bodywork is an indispensable support in dropping extra. It's a vehicle that could bring you to the taste of *I exist*. When you exist, when you know it by taste, doing Breema bodywork is sacred. Everything you do is sacred, because the emanation of what *is* is in it.

The present is the only reality, the only thing you can know for certain. When you are present, you have confidence in your True nature. You're connected to the bigger picture.

The universe functions according to the
Nine Principles of Harmony.
These principles are in you — not in the
outer aspect of yourself,
not in what you think you are,
but in your actual Self.

What does Body Comfortable mean? We have an approximate, relative meaning for every word and idea in our lives. We measure what is comfortable against something that is uncomfortable. So we know what's relatively more comfortable.

But the Nine Principles are not rooted in the relative. They enter into the relative, but their root is in Timelessness, in the Absolute, in Unity. Comfort is a dimension of Consciousness where everything is organized and working in harmony with our Timeless nature. To be in that dimension of Consciousness is to be truly comfortable. Of course, any degree of Body Comfortable is also of value. But now and then, it's good to remember that all the principles are Timeless. You can never master them, but you can walk toward them. Each principle is like an endless mountain whose peak you can never reach. Yet while you are climbing it, you experience the peak. Every step toward the principle guides you toward becoming present. Being present also has degrees. The more present you become, the more you taste something in yourself that is not thoughts and not feelings. With increasing receptivity, you move closer to your Timeless nature.

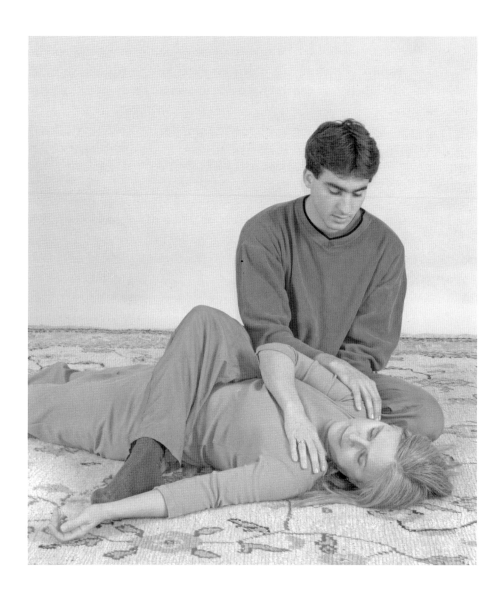

If you open any of the Nine Principles, you'll see the exact same shining truth in each one. You can find footprints of the ultimate intelligence in them. That's why you can never understand them fully. They aren't something to be understood. They are what you really are. At the same time, you can travel with them, taking step after step through your desire to understand. But your only chance for understanding them is while you are manifesting them in your life. At the moment you're actually working with Single Moment/Single Activity, you may get a glimpse of what Single Moment/Single Activity means. It's the same with all the other principles.

To practice Firmness and Gentleness, don't try to be firm. Don't try to be gentle. You only need to be present. Then firmness and gentleness manifest in harmony, because you are present. The "you" that you think you are is isolated. But the you that can be present is in unity, because whatever is present relates to everything that is present. In fact, the present is you, yourself. Your image, the person you imagine you are, lives in the past and future. But you yourself are always present.

When we practice Breema with the Nine Principles in the background supporting us, Breema becomes what it really is—a unifying method to first bring our mind, body, and feelings together, and then bring us to the unity of Knowledge and Being. Each grain of understanding so created connects us a little more with our Self and with everything that exists. That connection frees us from imaginary separation, and brings us to the grace of unity, which gives us a real taste of life.

In the entire universe,
there is no extra.

What if you make it your aim to live your life without extra? It doesn't matter, at first, how much you understand what the principle of No Extra means. Whatever you understand is enough to start with. Working with it simplifies you enough to move towards the real meaning of it.

You have thoughts while you're doing things. Are those thoughts extra? You have feelings. Your body has sensations. There is tension. Are these extra? Surprisingly, they are not! But if you take those thoughts, those feelings, or the body to be you, that identification is extra! Your identification with those thoughts is extra. So actually, only identification is extra, because life is that which is happening. Life is a process and it's constantly manifesting.

But we never seem to appreciate the flow of life. We drink buttermilk and say, "I wish this were tea." And when we drink tea, we say, "If only this were buttermilk." We create problems for ourselves by not being with what is. And to be with what is, we need to be present.

Extra is anything that's in the past or future. In the present, there is no extra.

You can also see extra in how you look at yourself. "I am good. I am busy." Whatever you say about yourself, whatever you add onto "I am" is extra. Because you are identified with the activity or description, and you unconsciously assume "I" means the vague and limited self-concept you hold in your mind.

If first you drop the description, you have a chance to taste what *I am* really means. *I am* is *I am* in the Totality, inseparable from the whole. *I am* in the moment. *I am*—free from name, shape, color, free from thoughts, feelings, and sensations. All those are functions. But *I am* is a statement of Existence. In *I am*, you have a chance to taste your existence in this very moment. That is freedom.

*Full Participation
simply means
Being-participation.*

To experience what taste is, work with the Nine Principles. Take one principle and work with it for a week. What does No Hurry/No Pause really mean? Work with it for a whole week. Not only when you're practicing Breema or Self-Breema. Work with it when you're in the kitchen cooking, when you walk, when you talk, when you shake hands, when you wash dishes, when you sweep. Then you see this is not a concept. It's a definite experience you come to for yourself.

By working with the principles yourself, you can experience something real, something beyond your conditioning. You can enter a new world—the world of direct knowing, the world of Being-participation, the world of meaning and purpose. Through the principles, you enter the present, and you find your inner atmosphere, your connection to reality.

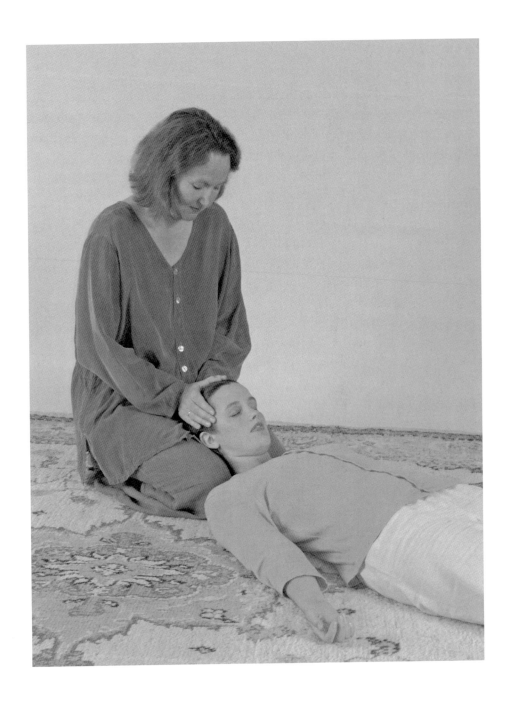

We need a way to come to reality. Breema starts with the body, because it's the simplest way. You have your body's weight to help you, and you have its breathing process. Connecting to those, you can come to the actual taste of *there is a body*. This taste is not the body, and it isn't really dependent on the body. Taste is your entrance into reality.

And reality always is. You may not always be available to receive it, but it's always there. Coming to your breathing, or to your body, is not an end in itself. It's a way to come to taste. The taste is not a taste of breath or of body—it's your consciousness becoming conscious of its own existence. Breathing is an event, a temporary event. But when you are conscious of events, your consciousness receives its light from Awareness, which is not an event.

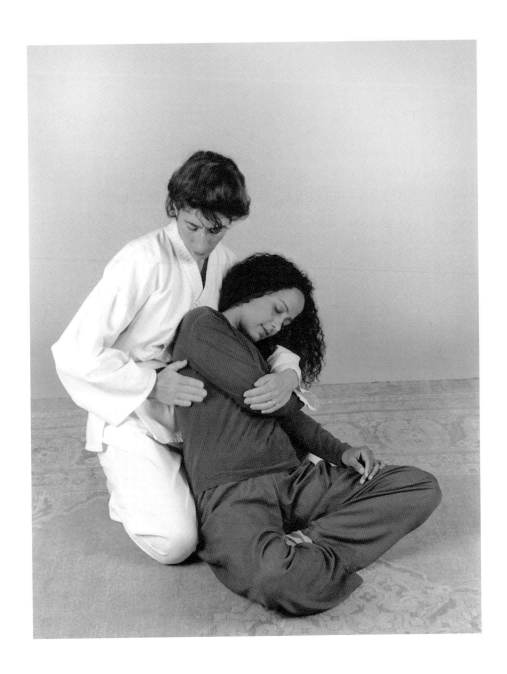

When you practice Breema bodywork with someone, the only thing you need is to be present. The sequences are a support for you to become open and receptive, so you can experience the taste of being present. When you become present, your True nature is emanating, and in that emanation, you and the recipient become united in a single field of acceptance. Your Timeless reality enters into time, and gives you the taste of *I exist*.

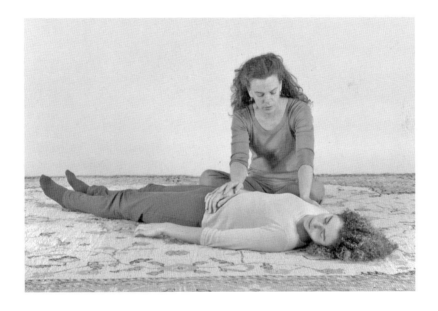

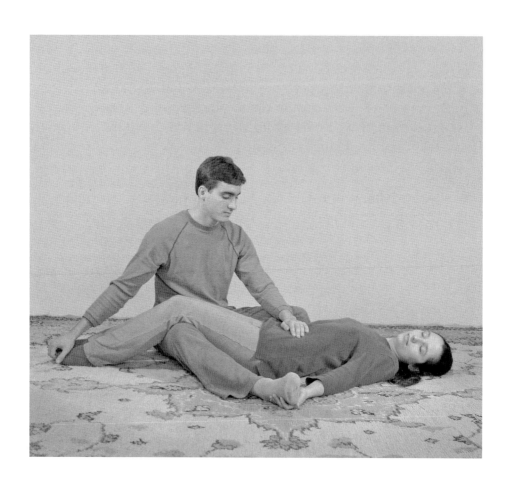

Our minds have been "educated" to record, retrieve, compare, and classify information. But when we repeat what we've heard or read, our words are hollow, because we don't really know what we're talking about! We don't experience an inner satisfaction when we mechanically present our mind's accumulated information as something we actually know, because that information hasn't become part of our *Being*.

When the mind becomes interested in registering the activity of our own body, we have more energy, because instead of separating itself from our body, the mind starts to participate in our body's activity. As we continue to register our body's manifestations with interest, our feelings start to participate, too, and we experience a new quality of aliveness.

When an Inner Authority is created through the unification of our body, mind, and feelings, and through our desire for Self-understanding, an impression of Existence is simultaneously received in all three. In fact, this *I* exists in the absence of thoughts and feelings. At the presence of that authority, we are connected to Existence. We remain ordinary, but life "tastes" different—the taste of I-AMness is in it.

"Do you know what freedom is?" someone once asked me. "I thought I did," I said, "until you asked." *Everything* in life is like that. At first, we assume we know about everything. But when that authority which knows you have a body exists, you have freedom from conceptual existence.

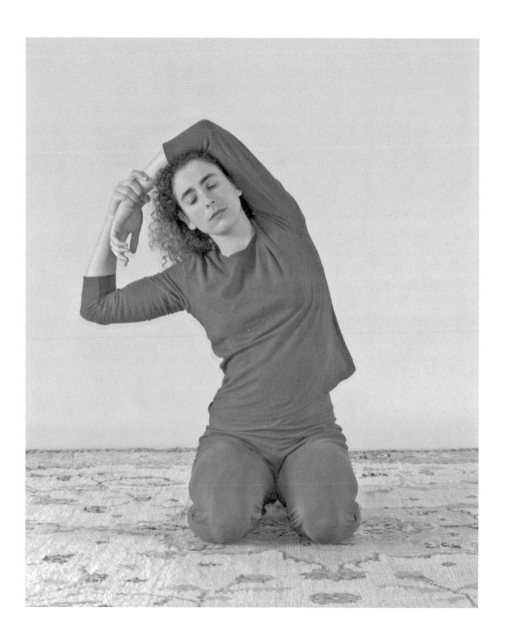

Breema can relax us, but that's not its principal aim. Breema decrystallizes the body, mind, and feelings.

As the body is decrystallized, it becomes capable of having new movements and postures. Its relationship to the life force changes.

As the feelings are decrystallized, they no longer swing between like and dislike. Instead, they respond to life directly.

As the mind is decrystallized, mind, feelings, and body can have a new relationship and function cooperatively.

Breema's principles don't say your mind or feelings have to be a certain way. Breema is simply a way of freeing energy for productive work. Whatever you wish to do, you need energy to do it. Associative mind, reactive feelings, and tense body waste energy. Working with the principles creates receptive mind, supportive feelings, and relaxed body. The energy that is usually consumed by the conflict between mind and feelings, and by physical tension, becomes available.

Doing Breema, doing Self-Breema, and applying any of the Nine Principles in your daily life—these support you to become present and remain present.

When you are present, others are supported to be present, and there is Mutual Support.

Any time you give support, Mutual Support is taking place, because you are receiving support simultaneously. Whenever you are in a position to give support, it's because you have been supported to be able to be in that position. At any moment you manifest in harmony with your understanding, in harmony with your Conscience, in harmony with your True nature, you are being supported.

When you recognize any phenomenon without commentary, Mutual Support is taking place. Say you have recognition of your body breathing. Where did you get this body? How is it able to breathe? The more you look, the more you see you are constantly receiving the support of Existence, every moment of your life.

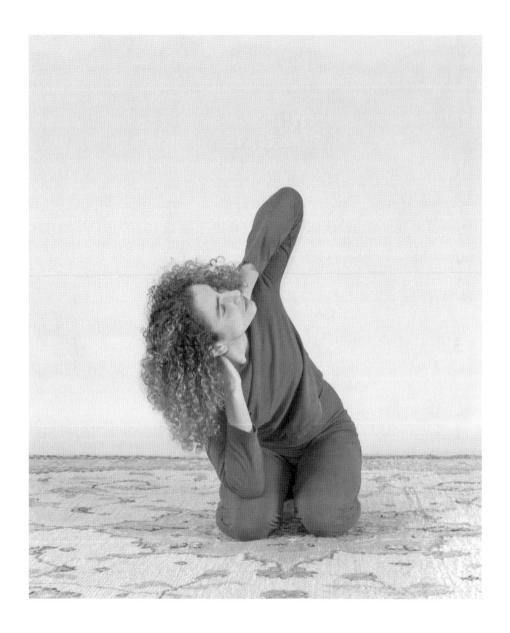

Coming to the present is not a technique. There's no technique that can bring you to be present for a moment. Techniques belong to the mind, and the mind is never present. It's always in the past or future.

That's why Breema is not a technique. Everything it has, even the specific sequences and Self-Breema exercises, are expressions of one universal energy. When you're connected to that, whatever you do is Breema. The activity of the body while you are present is Breema.

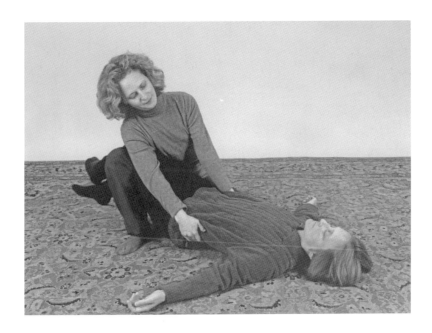

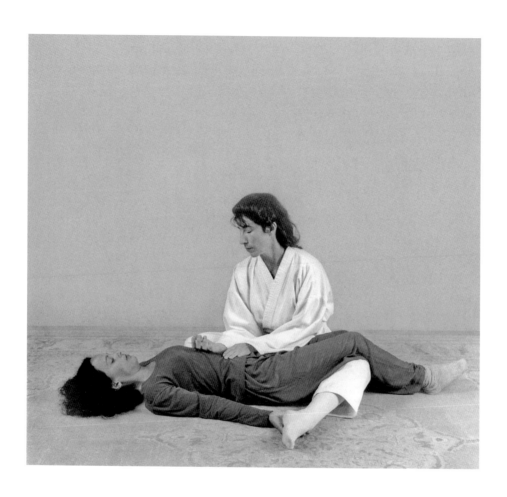

Four of the Nine Principles of Harmony start with "no"—No Extra, No Hurry/No Pause, No Force, and No Judgment. If you try to apply these four principles in your life, you'll soon find out that you are always using force in everything you do. You're always rushing, or caught in the dilemma of pausing. You're always judgmental about everyone and everything around you. And whatever you do, a lot of extra goes with it.

If you can see that that's the way you actually live your life, you have a new problem—how to see it nonjudgmentally. That means bringing it to acceptance. Not kicking an apple tree to try to make it produce oranges. This is how things are. First you have to see by your own observation that this is how you live your life, beyond the shadow of a doubt.

Breema doesn't tell you to fix what you see, because you can't. Breema points you to a dimension in yourself that is free of extra, of hurry and pause, of force, and of judgment. You can't come to this new dimension by educating your mind. You need a new education, one that helps you lose everything you've imagined yourself to be. You lose all the labels you've acquired—doctor, engineer, teacher—and at the same time, you lose your slavery to your thoughts and beliefs.

This new education is education through *taste*. Taste comes from Being. It's the entrance to what you really are, to who the universe intended you to be. Taste connects you to unity, and in unity, God and man are not separated. You can find awareness of that unity in yourself.

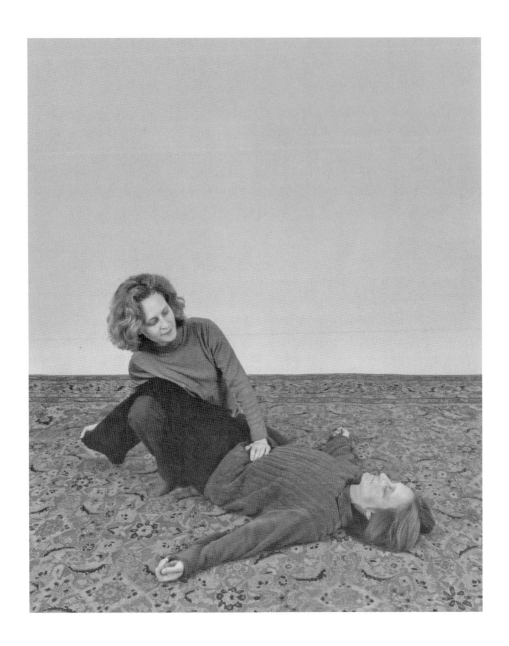

oment after moment, the universe comes into existence without force. Things in their natural state don't exert force. Whenever you use force, you create resistance. If you work with force, you become manipulative. And that makes people close up to you. We may think that by manipulating others we gain something, but we never do. We lose something.

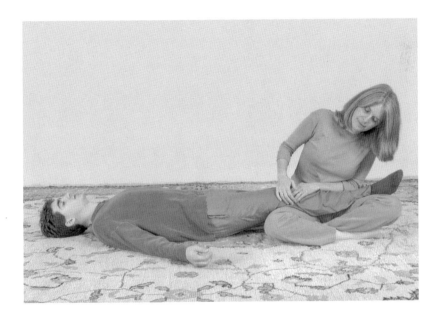

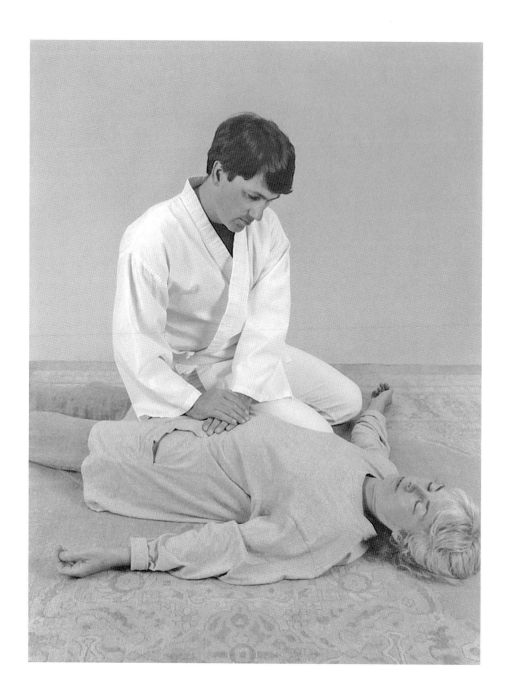

There is no reason to hurry, unless you project an outcome in the future—something you want that you don't have yet, or that hasn't happened yet. There is no reason to pause, unless you want to postpone the future loss of something you have now, or postpone an anticipated outcome. So we hurry and pause because we feel pressured by time.

Your body breathes. Your body has weight on the ground. The activity of the body takes place in the present. When your hand touches something, that's the only moment that exists. There is no "moment ago," when your hand was somewhere else. There's no "next moment," when your hand will be somewhere else. Everything you've done in your whole life is expressed in this one touch.

This is exactly how Existence manifests. In every moment the entirety is manifesting, every subatomic particle is manifesting. If you put time and space in the background, there is freedom from the measurement they create. Everything simply is as it is, unseparated from the Totality. Everything is an expression of the Totality. A drop of water is a representative of the entire ocean. If you take it separately, it loses that quality. You are a drop of water in Existence. When you take yourself separately, you're no longer a representative of the Totality. Existence manifests itself in unity. That's why there is No Hurry/No Pause. Because everything you do is really being done by Existence itself. Existence is manifesting itself.

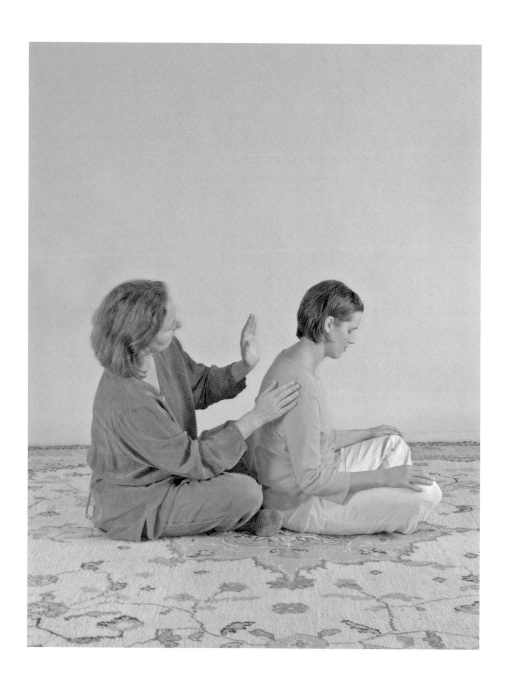

There is no extra in the universe. Everything enters into existence moment after moment, without any force. By its very nature, Existence has no judgment. Everything has its own right place, without hurry and without pause. When we're connected to our True nature, whatever we do is a single activity in a single moment. Gentleness and firmness are simultaneous expressions of the harmony of Existence. All things are in a mutually supportive relationship with each other. The body of the universe is comfortable, because all things are accepted as they are in the universal field.

The past and future are contained in the present, the present in the moment, and the moment is all there is. And that's the nature of reality. In this one complete, comprehensive universe, everything has room to grow, and so, the principle of constant change. Nothing can remain as it is. Moment after moment, everything changes and shows its temporary nature. Yet the permanent aspect is eternally present, always and everywhere. You are connected to the entire cosmos. All you need is to be present in yourself, and receive this blessing of infinite magnitude. You are as you are. Through acceptance of that, you connect to the bigger picture, where your *I* is permanent, immortal, unchanging. Every moment, you have a chance to enter into the taste of *I exist.*

To become more and more present,
do whatever you are doing
with Full Participation.
Every activity is a gift
if you do it willingly
and with Full Participation.

We are affected by our upbringing, by our education, and by all the influences that surround us, from the media to everything we see or touch. Each has an impact on us, and these influences are always there.

Because of these influences, we relate to everything we see associatively. We filter everything through this mechanical consciousness and then what we do is always dictated by these previous influences.

But the reality of your life, what you could actually call your life, is only in the present. When the present moment is lost, you're not living your life, you're living your conditioning.

If you agree with this without proving or disproving it for yourself, it just becomes another layer of conditioning. Anything you accept without verifying becomes more conditioning. Even if it's all true, it doesn't help you.

Working with the Nine Principles and practicing Breema until you "get Breema in your body" gives you the possibility to create a new relationship to life, one that doesn't stem from your conditioning. Every moment you have of being present becomes the foundation of that relationship. Those moments organize you inside, and create an atmosphere that's free from past and future, free from your conditioning. When you connect to that atmosphere, you find yourself having new thoughts, new feelings, and a new posture toward life.

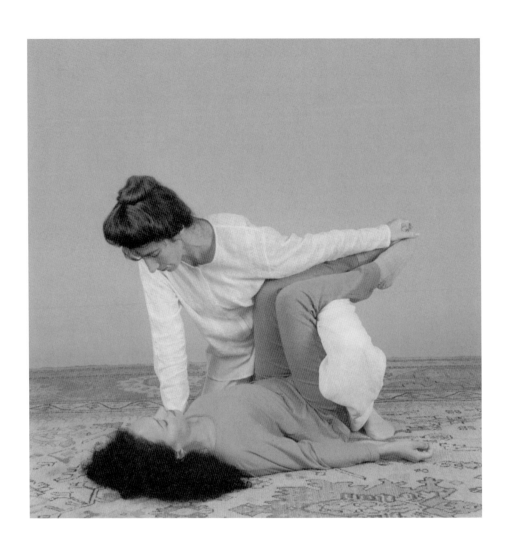

If I ask my mind to help me practice Full Participation, something extra always comes in. The mind starts to analyze and comment and judge. But there is one thing that brings *less* instead of extra—the mind can stay with the process of inhalation and exhalation. To support that, I start doing Breema to get the help of my body. I lean in, and exhale. As I release, I inhale. Now my mind doesn't travel to the past and future, because it's got a job to do. When the mind and body work together and stay together for a while, at some point I experience the presence of a new energy, which comes from the participation of the feelings. Now I am connected to life. Because when body, mind, and feelings are united in an activity, something else becomes present—a messenger from my True nature. Then I am connected to the bigger picture.

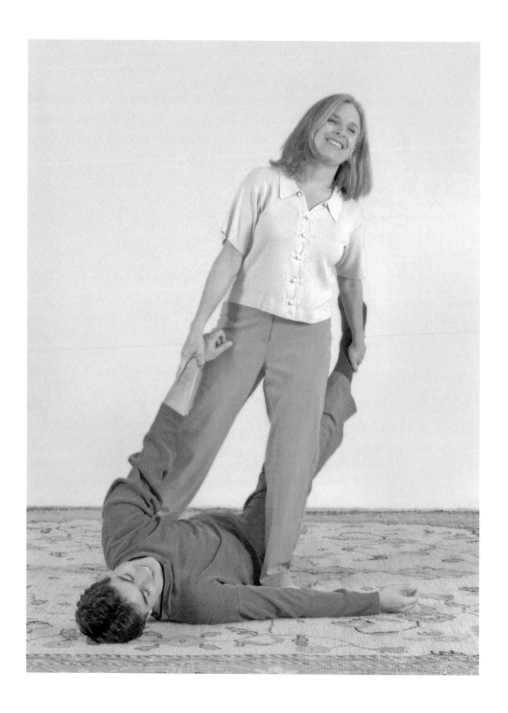

We do not know our true feelings, but we do know how to nurture them. When our mind and body work as a unit, and in harmony with each other, we clear the ground for this nurturing process to take place. Then many things support and nurture our feelings.

Our feelings are nurtured:

When we are present in our daily activities,

When we are less judgmental,

When we have acceptance of ourselves and the people around us,

When we do things with attention and use our abilities to their maximum,

When we willingly do something that needs to be done,

When we make ourselves available to the needs of our friends and neighbors,

When we have a sense of a greater Existence than ourselves, and in our actions and activities we carry that sense with us,

When we practice forgiveness,

When we wish not to think negatively about the people we come in contact with,

When we allow the simple pleasures of life to be fully appreciated,

When we live our life with gratitude for that which is given to us,

When we acknowledge that we are being helped by what's been set up in our surroundings,

When we remember how dear our parents are, and how much we owe to them,

When we wish to support everyone we're supported by,

When we acknowledge and respect the good deeds of others,

When we are willing to pay for what we receive,

When we have a sense of gratitude for our daily accomplishments,

When we appreciate that which is,

When our words and thoughts about others are sincere,

When we train ourselves to do small things for the welfare of our planet and humanity,

When we use things correctly and avoid misusing them,

When we shake hands with a friend while connected to our body,

When our mind is receptive while listening,

When we appreciate nourishment more than stimulation,

When we wish to take good care of ourselves, simply and effectively,

When we don't take advantage of the misfortune of others,

When we remember the temporariness of the life of the body,

When we relate to each occasion as if it's the only time we have,

When we live each day as if it's the only day we have left to live,

When we live less and less in our mind, and recognize that we're surrounded by life,

When we appreciate the good in others, and see their shortcomings simply as a lack of knowledge and experience in some particular area, rather than as faults,

When we have room to see opposing sides at the same time,

When we have a small goal to accomplish each day and we have well-wishing for ourselves to accomplish it,

When we remember that life has meaning,

When we wish this meaning to reveal itself to us,

When we pray nonverbally,

When our posture toward life is humble and has dignity,

When we say "yes" and when we say "no," not out of weakness,
but from our knowing,

When we look at money as energy and energy as money,
and we use them wisely,

When we treat others as we wish to be treated,

When we respect others' belongings and accomplishments and
have well-wishing for them,

When we wish to say that which we know, and avoid saying what we
don't know,

When we respect simplicity more than complication.

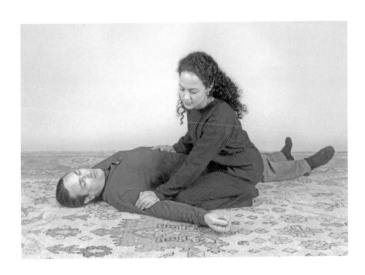

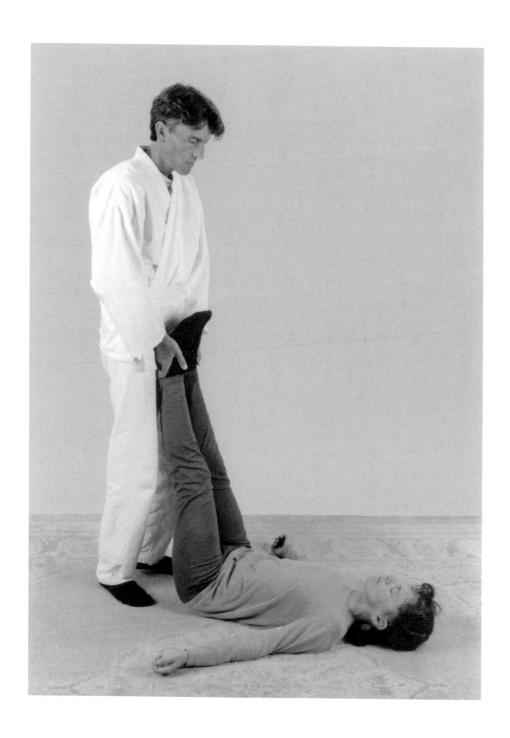

In order to verify the truth of what we think, we need the assistance of our feelings and our body. That which we think must also be felt and sensed simultaneously.

We support this process by giving the mind one simple job to do, asking it to receptively *register* our own body's weight and breathing.

At first, we find this challenging—our mind has long been accustomed to being our "boss." It repeatedly wants to return to its world of imagination and useless wandering, and shuffle and reshuffle the information it has received from the outside, falsely labeling it as knowledge and sometimes even as understanding. The misuse of the meaning of knowledge and understanding keeps us more at the periphery of the mind, and invites our mechanicality to further dominate us.

Partial knowledge is complex.
Total knowledge is simple.

The person who has real understanding
is very simple.

The person with partial understanding
is complicated.

So whenever we recognize that we are again lost in our thoughts, we simply ask our mind to return to its new job and remain with it until we experience the presence of a new energy which we call *Being-presence*. Then, once again, our three aspects are actively participating in life.

Slowly, we become familiar with the distinctive *taste* that's present when our mind is registering the body at the presence of the feelings.

These are not the feelings we are familiar with, which work only via attraction and repulsion. These true feelings are simply *present*.

This is our direction. The mind does not *think* about the body's weight and breath, it *registers* the body's weight and breathing. This registration is the receptive quality of mind that we are after—it takes place in the *absence* of thought. When the mind is receptive, we *experience* that which it registers. When mind, feelings, and body all experience the fact of *there is a body,* our experience becomes more definite knowledge, and we have less identification. Then, when we have essential questions about the purpose and meaning of our lives, we have a base. Instead of entertaining these questions abstractly, we may seek knowledge that we can verify through our actual experience, through *taste,* rather than settling for theories to believe in.

Once our mind "settles into" a correct relationship with the feelings and the body, it could, with their support, think intentionally, ponder, and reason soundly. That's why our aim is to bring the mind, feelings, and body to work together.

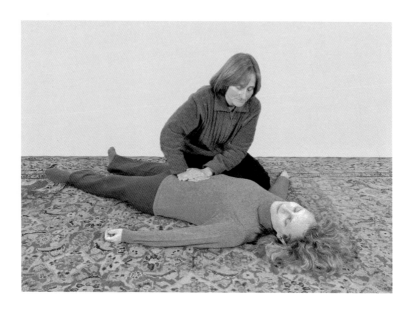

Energy is flowing
through the entire universe all the time.
In the first second you place your hand
on the recipient's body,
that energy is there, provided you don't
block it with your thoughts and ideas.
Then your touch has all
the Nine Principles in it, with
no expectation and no preconception.

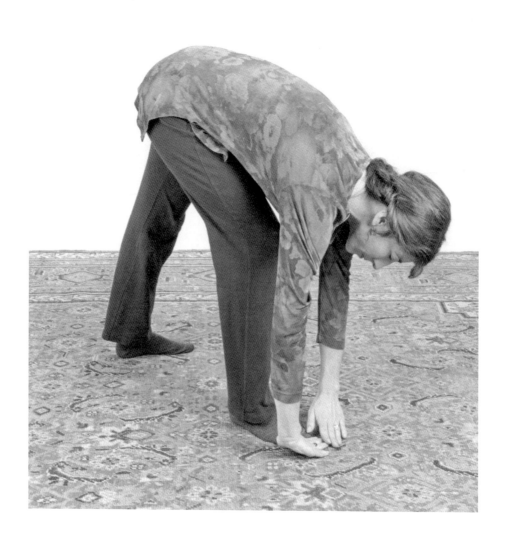

How can I connect? My mind is in a thousand different places. I can't connect, because the traffic in my mind doesn't let me. So, I ask my mind to register inhalation and exhalation. If I do that, and keep with it, something happens. The traffic decreases. The more I stay with my breath and my body, the less traffic there is. In some moment, there is no traffic. I am present. I am connected.

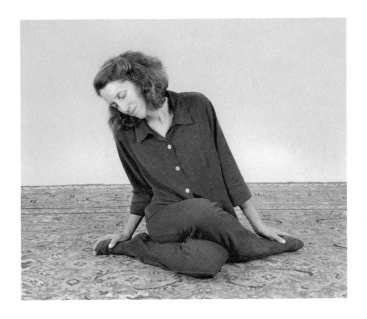

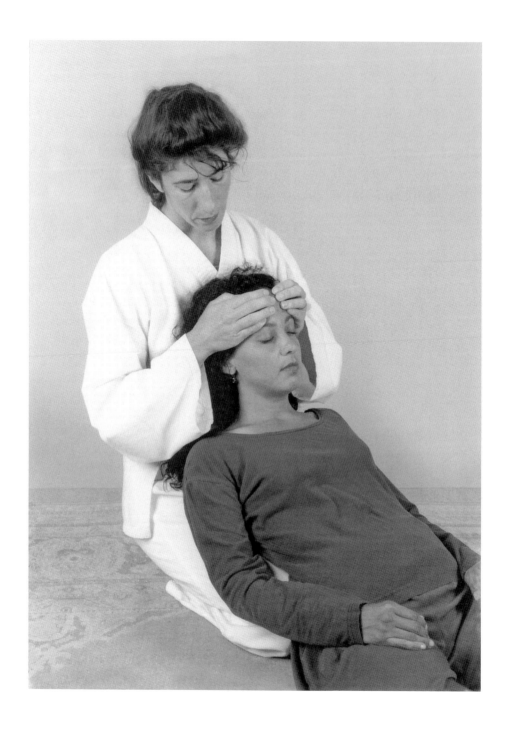

Single Moment/Single Activity means entering into diversity without losing your connection to Unity. Single Moment and Single Activity can't be separated. They are simultaneous, not sequential. The Absolute and its emanation are simultaneous. We manifest in time and space, but the reality of our existence is beyond time and space, in Unity, in eternity. Nothing is separated. If you are a reflection of reality, that reflection is part of reality, not something separate that needs to be erased. Once you see that, you understand that everything belongs, all your "good" and "bad" attributes and experiences, because life is that which is happening.

How can you have a single moment? You have to be free of the past and free of the future. Otherwise, your past associations and expectations of the future enter, and instead of a moment, you are lost in a conceptual relationship to time.

When you are present, there is a single moment. Your receptivity to the moment becomes a single activity. In the absence of thoughts and feelings, you enter into the present, and there is one moment and one activity.

Existence has four levels:
matter, energy, Consciousness,
and Awareness.

Matter, energy, and Consciousness
have no independent existence;
they are simply Awareness manifested.

We relate to the body through thoughts and sensations. That's why we can never understand it. We're always confused by it. We're always worried about it.

But there is a reality that is higher than what our mind and senses tell us. In this dimension, Consciousness is the authority, not our mind. And Consciousness tells us that the body is made of light. It is vibration. If we look at the body as light and vibration, we are closer to the reality of it, because the real body is permanent. It is eternal. We no longer need to worry about the body. Instead, we can appreciate it. Then we don't look at our hand as an object, attached to the body, which we also relate to as just another object. We see it as something that's connected to the entire cosmos. Light is connected to all light. We can see the body as a truly beautiful phenomenon, because we relate to it in a real way.

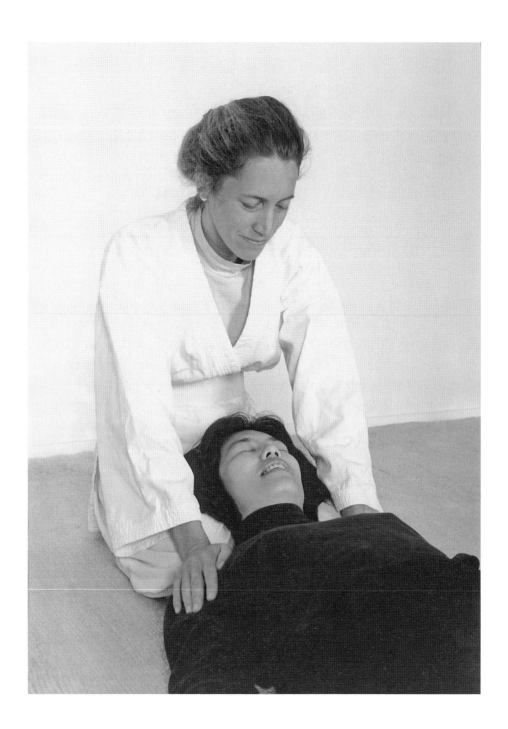

Practicing Breema, there's no description of what your hand is touching. Your hand is there, and whatever takes place, takes place there. You are there *with* your hand, so that "there" and "here" are one. No part of you needs to hold itself separate to describe from the sidelines the sensations of warmth or cold, softness or hardness. They are, whatever they are. In Full Participation, there is no need for description. You could talk about the recipient's body till doomsday, but it is what it is. Description neither adds nor subtracts. It only confuses us, and shifts the emphasis away from knowing ourselves.

At the same time, our minds have been thinking and describing for nearly our entire lives. Should we try to stop it while we're practicing Breema? Why not let it do what it always does? You don't have to involve yourself with it. Whatever sensation your hand feels, and whatever description your mind gives to it, there's no problem. You don't have to be with that. Thoughts come and go. You don't need to be inside those thoughts. Prior to thinking is *being*. You *exist*, prior to thought. Because a thought comes, it doesn't mean you have to lose your connection to your *Being*, to Existence, and get involved in the thought. Then you're no longer here.

Let thoughts come, let thoughts go. Let feelings come, let feelings go. Let sensations come, let sensations go. They are just temporary manifestations of our real nature.

There is one Awareness,
one Consciousness, one energy,
***one** Existence.*

The purpose of practicing Breema is to come to the present, to the taste of being present. That's where you actually taste your own existence. Breema is about that *actually*—

> Being
> > Right now
> > > Everywhere
> > > > Every moment
> > > > > Myself
> > > > > > Actually.

Nothing is actual until you taste it. So you come to the body, come to your breathing, to the process of inhaling and exhaling, until that traffic that's always inside your mind slows down. At some point, the traffic stops for a moment, and you come to your own mind. Your essential mind. The unconditioned mind. With that mind supporting you, you can really practice the Nine Principles. Then it may even become possible for you to find your true identity.

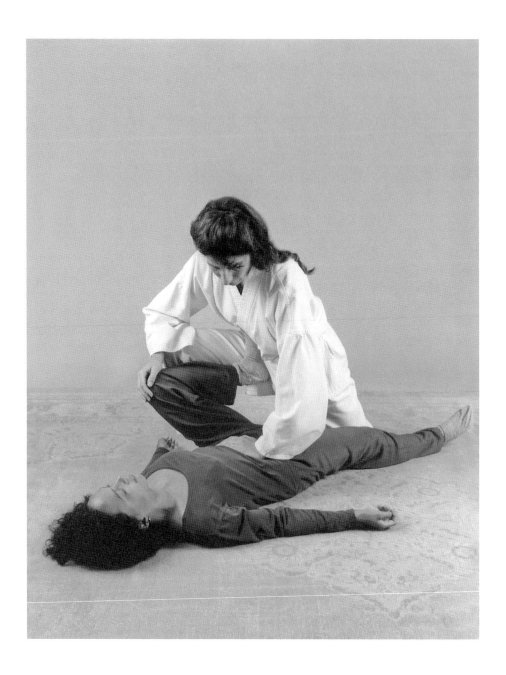

You cannot separate Breema bodywork or Self-Breema from the background of Breema. The background is Breema's philosophy. There is one unified Existence. So when you practice, the entirety is with you. When you're here, it's not some little "here." You are in a space that is spaceless, in time that is Timeless, in your real body, which is without boundaries. You're in Existence, which is the Totality. These are not words to say to yourself, not thoughts to think. This is a posture toward Existence. When this is your posture, then you brush, and everything is brushing with you. You bend, and everything is bending with you. The entirety is moving. When you tap, it's not you doing something by yourself. Existence is expressing itself, your Timeless nature is being expressed. The past disappears. It's nothing but a concept. In each moment, all of the Nine Principles are being expressed, and you can't separate any one of them from the rest.

There is only one body,
and no matter where you touch,
you're touching the whole body.

The body is universal. It functions with
the principle of inner connectedness.
Every cell is blessed with
total knowledge of the whole,
and so is always in unity with it.

Body breathes, body has weight on the ground. This is the cornerstone of practicing Breema. Because you can't say your body had weight a minute ago. You can't say your body is going to have weight a minute from now. Having weight means you *experience* it. Only then can you truthfully say it. That's how you enter the world of reality. You say what you experience, because then it's real for you.

So while you're doing Breema with someone (or doing any activity in daily life), experience body breathes, body has weight. *Your* body. Because that's the one you can taste. This moment is for this moment. You don't need to try to "collect" it, so you can remember it in the next moment. This moment is this moment. Finished. You are where you are. The next moment has no connection to the previous one. Things aren't connected by time and space. They're connected by reality, and reality is free from time and space, and is in this moment.

That's how it is with Breema. You can't understand any of the Nine Principles through words. Only when you have a taste of one of them do you know what it is. In fact, the principles make you free from your ideas. You put your hands on the recipient's body, without ideas. That means you're not inside your head, you're not at the mercy of your thoughts. Life is manifesting. Life is as it is. Can you change it? You can't. But you can taste it, you can experience it. Then you are alive in your life.

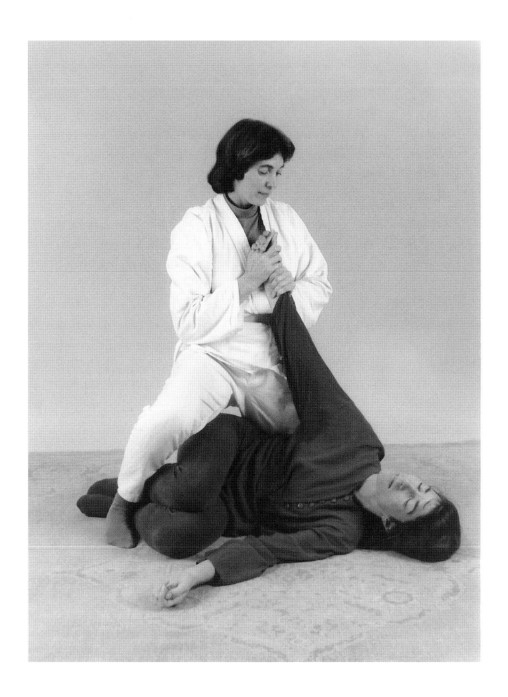

When you practice Breema bodywork, your body is manifesting. You are working with the recipient's body, but that's not what it's all about. During the session, acceptance slowly comes in. At some point, you let go of the concept of practitioner and recipient, and then there's an atmosphere of life giving to life.

The flexibility you gain from Breema doesn't come from stretching. It comes from inner receptivity, it comes from your new understanding, it comes from actualizing the Nine Principles in your life. When you are present, you are in harmony with your True nature, with the entirety. You receive Conscious energy in your body. Then, you have the sensitivity, the receptivity to know what you need, to know how to move through life and grow in wisdom and sincerity.

*The Nine Principles are not
something you can master,
because each principle is endless.
But because the principles
are directional, your understanding
grows as you work with them.*

Firmness and Gentleness are never separate. They are always together, two necessary aspects of one energy and one reality. They complement each other.

In Firmness and Gentleness we can find the possibility to harmonize our mental and emotional activity, so they can support each other. Then we can feel what we think, and think what we feel. We can know the quality of our thoughts, and see whether or not there is any truth in them, or whether they have nothing to do with reality.

Our ordinary feelings are emotional reactions to our thoughts. Our real feelings are something entirely different. They neither like nor dislike. They have one aim—to be present, and support the activity of our mind in the direction of becoming conscious.

Practicing Breema, firmness and gentleness can be simultaneously present. You receive an impression of yourself, and you express what you've received. While being totally gentle, you express the firmness that comes from understanding yourself, from knowing where you are and what you're doing. In short, Firmness and Gentleness guides you toward being present, toward becoming yourself, free from past and future, so you can live your life in harmony with all that exists.

Inhalation and exhalation are two aspects of one process, one energy. They can help you stay on the "tightrope" of being present. At any given moment you have a chance to experience body breathing— inhaling and exhaling. If you stay with this process of inhalation and exhalation, you can remain on the tightrope. There, you receive a taste, a taste of Existence, because the body is a connecting factor that connects you to everything that exists.

Breema looks at the body not only as matter and energy—it also relates to it as Consciousness and Awareness.

When there is a background of Existence, you exist. Your existence is given. Knowing that you exist is your *I*.

When there is a background of Consciousness, you know you have a body. Your body exists. When you look with your consciousness, whatever you look at exists. When you're in the mind, you can't do that, because the mind can't see. Seeing is always from a consciousness that is higher than what it looks at.

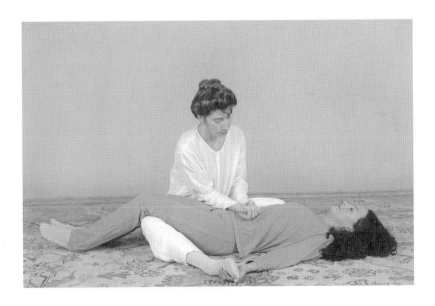

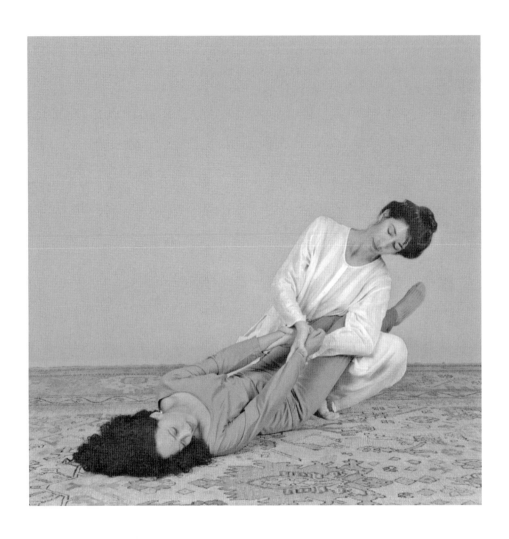

Single Moment/Single Activity—the whole truth is right there. In the moment, the *only* moment, the single moment, there is one *I*, the universal *I*, the *I* of Existence. This *I* manifests itself in a single activity—it expresses its *am-ness*. *I am.* This is the ultimate statement, the pure expression of something that exists. When the Timeless manifests in time, *I am.* When life expresses itself in form, *I am.* When God's presence is tasted by someone, *I am.* When your consciousness participates in your activity, *I am.* When your love of life is present even while you're ignorant, *I am.* When your understanding doesn't disappear even while you're confused, *I am.*

The art and intelligence of Existence shows itself in *I am.* Single Moment/Single Activity is the union of *I* and *am.* It's the union of your Timeless nature and your relative nature, the relationship between the Absolute and its emanation, the truth of all that exists. Everything in the universe announces this truth, moment after moment. It's the basis of the relationship between Awareness and its emanation of Consciousness, energy, and matter, down to the smallest subatomic particle.

As big as it is, Single Moment/Single Activity is simple. If you don't restrict it to your mind, but let it settle in your heart, then in *I am,* you express the love of Existence on the Earth. Because in *I am,* there is no separation. *I am* doesn't mean "I am, and you are not." *I am* means there is one total Existence manifesting.

Combinations of the levels of Consciousness, energy, and matter are all manifested Awareness.

Every time we receive a taste in our Being, we are seeing a part of the whole picture of Existence. We are a part in the Totality, in union with the whole Totality. We are a drop in the ocean, in union with the ocean. Consciousness sees and has tastes. Since what we see is only a part, our aim is to always come to a new taste, to new seeing, so we constantly expand and refine our organized picture of Existence. This process is endless, because there will always be a more complete understanding possible, no matter how many tastes we include to form our understanding.

After you've had a taste of *there is a body,* or a taste of being present, your mind may come in and question it. Let the mind come, let doubts come. What do they have to do with you? If you find a gold coin, and later your mind comes in and says, "You don't have any gold," you don't have to argue. You just put your hand in your pocket and touch the coin, or you take it out and look at it. Taste is in you. When doubts come, don't start arguing with your mind. Just come back to the taste.

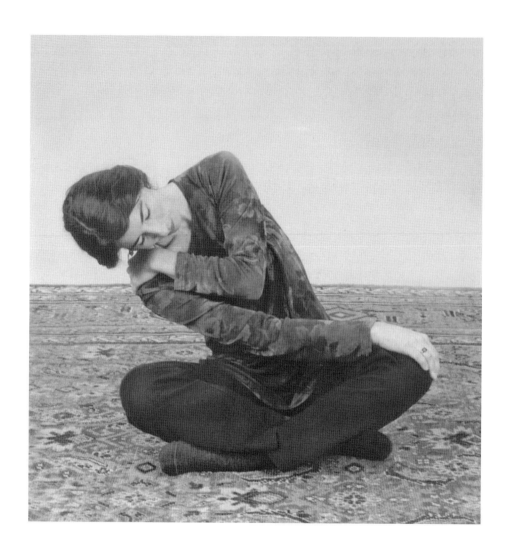

If you allow yourself, in this very moment, to be who you really are, then whatever you do is Breema. Because Breema is the expression of your True nature, moment after moment.

Of course there are many Breema sequences and Self-Breema exercises to practice. As a Breema student, you practice Breema bodywork and Self-Breema exercises to build a foundation that can help you come to the essence of Breema. They help you get a taste of what this is really about, so it doesn't remain theoretical for you.

Breema itself is not about the body, mind, emotions, or sensations. They're included, but the aim is Self-understanding. Self-understanding doesn't belong to time—it's not temporary. It belongs to the permanent dimension of Existence, and never disappears.

Information changes. New information supplants the old. Knowledge is information you have verified for yourself. And understanding is the union of Being and knowledge. Whatever you understand becomes an aspect of your permanent, eternal existence. The aim of Breema is Self-understanding, because by understanding yourself, you understand everything.

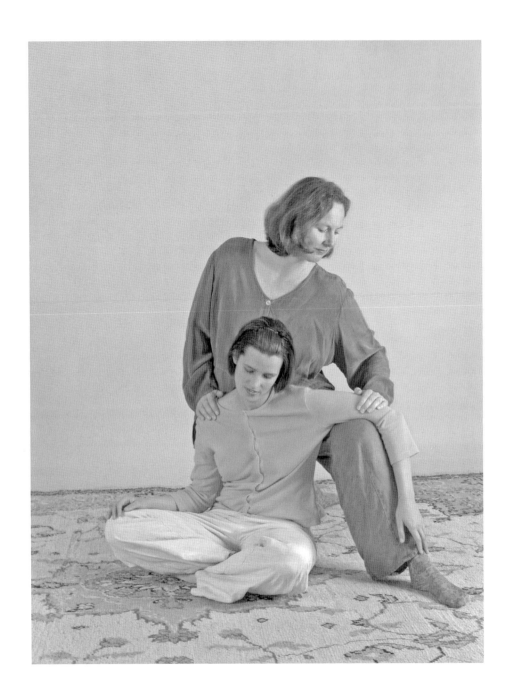

Three things are necessary. The first is to get a taste of being present. The second is to invite the present into your life, that is, to be present in daily life. The third is to remain present.

For the first part, learning and practicing Breema bodywork and the Nine Principles of Harmony help you. You discover that you are not just a head walking around on two legs, wearing a nametag. You have an opportunity to actually taste that *there is a body*. To taste that you are breathing. To support having a taste, you connect to the fact that the body breathes, the body has weight. As you *experience* these, your mind becomes less occupied, more available to you, more with the body.

Because otherwise, you are always thinking. You are always lost in thought, even when you think you're not thinking. By connecting to your breath and weight, you have a chance to see "there are thoughts, but they are not me." You and the process of thinking are not the same thing. You are wearing clothes, but you are not your clothes. You know that, because you put them on in the morning, and you take them off at night. You get in and out of your car. That's how you can tell that your car is not you. You go in and out of your house, so you can see that you're not your house. But thoughts are tricky. You don't see that you went into one, and came out and entered another thought. Because you have been thinking all the time, mechanically, habitually. The process just goes on by itself. But to *taste*, to actually experience what your body is doing, you have to become present.

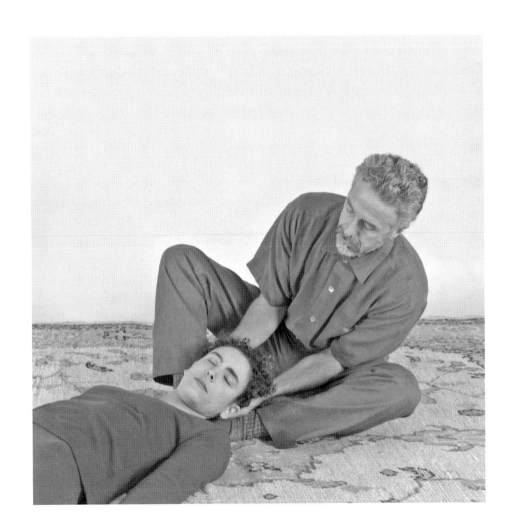

We need to come to the dimension of consciousness where we can see things as they are. The real is real. Thoughts are *about* the real, not the real itself. If you get caught in thoughts and take them to be real, you disappear. You don't exist anymore. You are a man or woman in the head. But you can come out of the jail of thought, via breath and weight of the body. Come out, into this moment of your existence.

Divine love is the reality of Existence, and it is flowing, moment after moment. But the mind has to open to Consciousness in order to receive this emanation. When you receive it, you know you exist, and that you are in unity with Existence. Nothing is separated. This is being present. You can't come to the present mentally. But working with the Nine Principles in daily life can help. When you taste that you are present, you *are*. You *exist*.

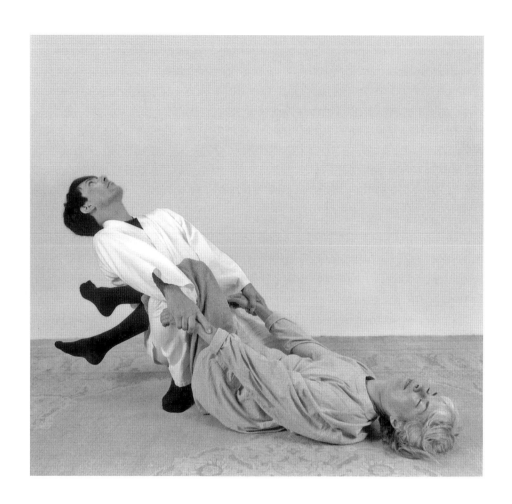

We don't really know who we are. But by working with the Nine Principles, and by practicing Breema and Self-Breema, you may get a taste of something that exists. Without the body, that something would not have a vehicle of expression, and you would never know about it. So the body is a vehicle that can connect you to reality. But if you just take the vehicle to be reality, you lose your connection to your True nature, which is eternal, not physical and temporary. Because of your eternal nature, your body becomes real, not the other way around! *You don't exist because of your body.* Because *you exist,* your body exists.

We think we are defined by this body, confined by our own skin. But this way of seeing ourselves is totally unexamined. If you could put on a pair of glasses that would let you see reality, you'd see that the body is just a tiny part of yourself, and is in you. You are not in it. You are not limited by time and space. In fact, you are not limited by anything! Your existence is universal. It's cosmic existence. That means the entirety, the whole of Existence is one. The essential reality of you and everyone else is one. That reality expresses itself in diversity, so we each have our unique qualities. You are you, and I am me, and there is countless diversity. When we come to the Timeless dimension, free from time and space, we enter into unity. Here, everything is one. If we relate to this from our thoughts, we mix up these dimensions. We relate to these properly only in our Being.

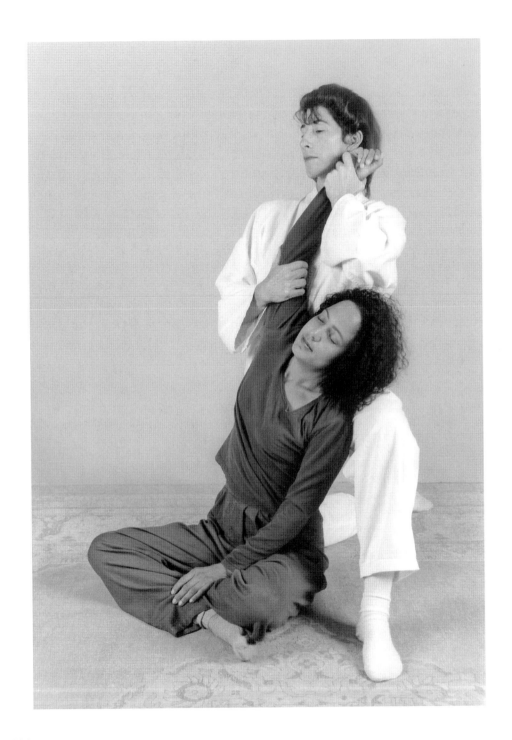

Receiving Breema, you can have a taste of being more yourself. You get a hint of what it means to be natural, to be connected. Of course, you're going to lose it. But you know you had that taste. Then, during the day, you can do one Self-Breema exercise, you can work with one of the Nine Principles, to come closer to that taste again. Because in the moment you have a taste of being present, you are free from the mind, free from past and future, and therefore free from your suffering.

It's not that we choose to be in the past or future. We do it automatically, out of habit. But each time we taste *I have a body*, we are present for a moment. The more we put this into practice, the more often we remember during our day that we wish to be present. And more often, we have a chance to *be*.

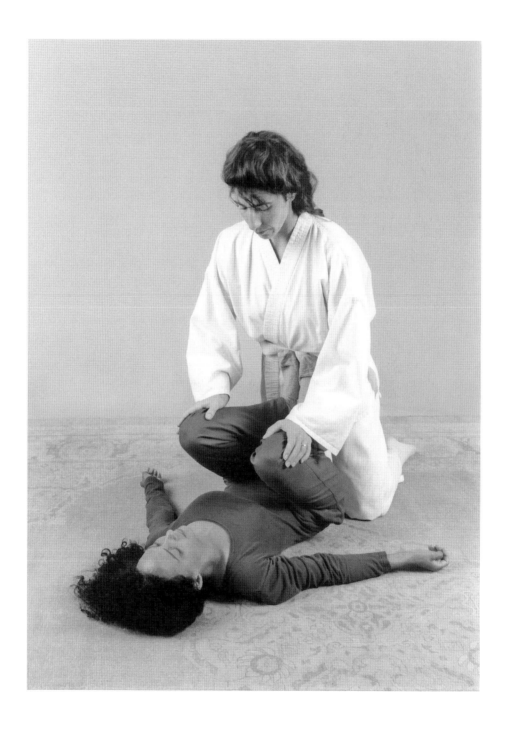

Without its background, Breema isn't really Breema. The background is part of placing your hand on the recipient's body. The more this background is *realized* by you, the more it becomes a part of you. The more Consciousness becomes a part of your cells, your bones, your hands, the more the emanation of your True nature is present. That's what makes Breema Breema. Doing Breema means letting the reality of who you really are manifest itself, moment after moment. It doesn't need explanation. So the aim of practicing Breema is simply to be present.

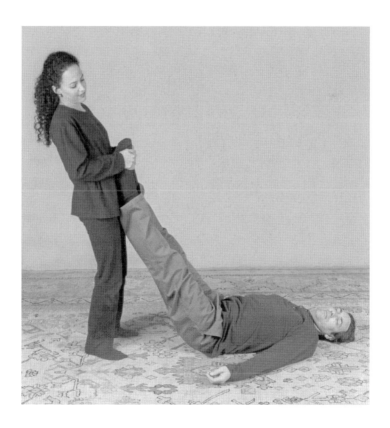

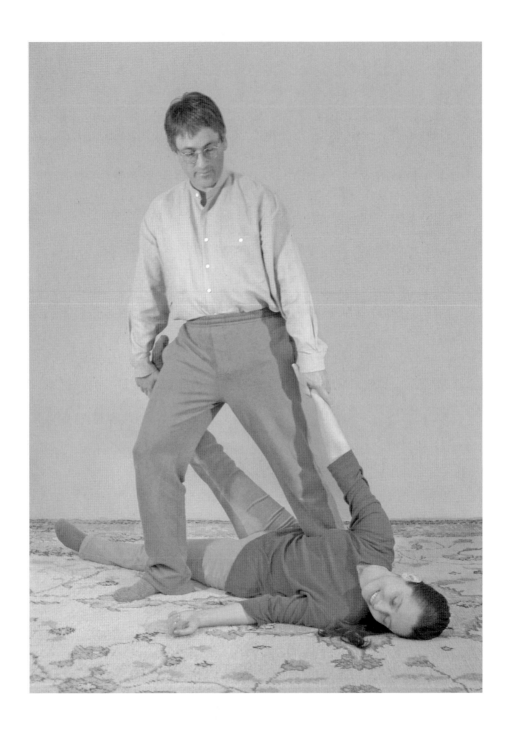

When you do Breema, of course there are sensations. Your hands are receiving sensory information. But you could receive that sensory input as an impression, without interpreting it. Then there are thoughts. Thoughts flow in and out, bringing many associations and images of the past and future. Your feelings are active too, coming and going, liking and disliking. And the body is doing Breema.

But all of this could take place in the background, while you have a consciousness that is not a thought, feeling, or sensation. That consciousness is *aware* of the thoughts, feelings, and sensations, but it does not identify with them. When this consciousness is present, you are present.

As you do Breema, let the joy
of Existence be present with you.
Be as simple as you can be.

There is no need for activity in your mind
and feelings. Drop all expectation.

And if you need to occupy your mind,
just registering the weight of the body and
the fact of inhalation and exhalation will do.

In the simplicity of Breema, there is unity, there is connectedness. Whenever you give someone a Breema bodywork session, you are giving Breema to yourself. But this self is unseparated. It means the entirety. You're not working on muscles and bones. You are inviting Conscious energy to manifest, and Conscious energy harmonizes us.

You don't need to think. You don't need to know what you're going to do. You don't need a self-image. You only need presence. You don't have to check by asking yourself "Am I present or not?" You start as if you are present. As you continue, your inner atmosphere becomes more and more available. It is both impersonal and personal. It is impersonal because it is universal. It is personal because you are emanating it. In fact, you are the emanator, the emanation, and the process of emanation—all three. Every particle in the universe in its natural state is that.

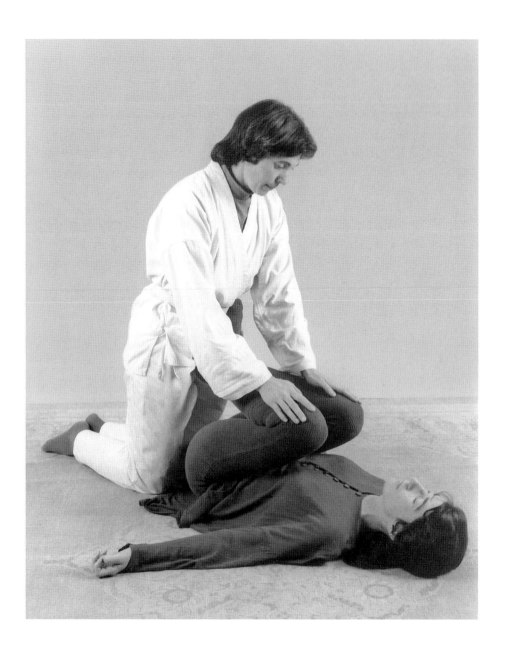

We understand money better than we understand energy. We know that we have to earn money and that it's best not to waste it. People who lack this simple clarity are always short of money and always have problems.

It's the same with energy. We need to receive it, and spend it wisely. But we seldom think of it like that. We accept that we happen to be here, haphazardly, and after seventy or eighty years, we're gone, so we try to "make the best of it."

If we see the importance of energy for our life, we may become interested in how to earn it, and how to spend it wisely. The first things we need to see are the areas in which we spend a lot of energy uselessly, without profit.

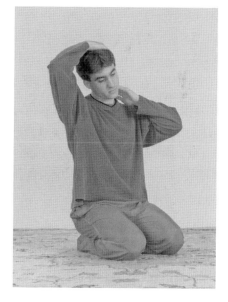

That's where Breema comes in. The wealth of vitality you feel after one Breema sequence is a result of your essential aspect receiving support. Breema is one whole. You can't really separate it into bodywork and philosophy. It's a whole package that makes you truly wealthy. If you work with any of the Nine Principles during the day, you have much more energy. We receive energy from food, drink, air, and impressions. But our energy reservoir is determined by our posture toward life, our attitude, the way we think about life, the way we feel about it, the way we sense it, the way we perceive it.

Breema's purpose is to bring us to a new way of thinking, a new way of feeling, to a new posture toward life. This is a new type of education, not education by words and concepts. This is education by *taste*. Taste nurtures your Being. And through your Being, you can receive Conscious energy, much finer than the energy you're used to. When you receive it, instead of thinking, you *realize*. Your realizations give you an inner organization. Look at how much energy you gain when you organize your desk. That's a fraction of what you gain when you organize your "inner desk." When your posture toward life is organized, you come to harmony with yourself, with your surroundings, with all life, and with Existence itself.

When you have a lot of organized energy, you don't waste so much. Wasting comes from an imbalanced state. You can see how much money people spend when they're emotionally disturbed.

Breema gives you a new education that you can verify for yourself. In fact, it's the self-verification that educates you. You can't receive it mentally. You have to get Breema in your body. When you get a taste of it in your body, then you really resonate with what you hear. Before that, you are not yourself. Your mind isn't your own mind. It's a conditioned mind, and you think and hear with it. Just as you can't put something in a room that's already filled up from floor to ceiling, you have to find an unconditioned part of yourself in order to receive knowledge that comes from an unconditioned source.

Breema bodywork and Self-Breema are important because they help your body become a vehicle that can receive Conscious energy. Once you are able to receive Conscious energy, you can receive more, because you have something that recognizes and appreciates it. In the same way, receiving Breema can give you tastes of the Nine Principles. Then when you hear about them, something in you knows what they are. They are no longer just attractive concepts.

*Our mind, by itself, cannot be
a source of understanding.*

*Understanding is the union
of sound knowledge and Being.*

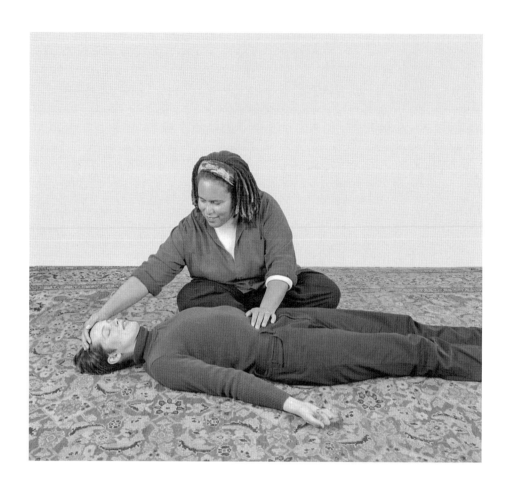

Deeper understanding comes directly from your Timeless nature. Your mind may receive it, but it can't hold onto it. So whenever you wish for truth, come back to your True nature, to the taste of Existence. Why search for the truth you received half an hour ago? Right now it's a new universe. Every moment is brand new. At the same time, if you connect to your body while your understanding is alive, you become more able to carry that understanding with you into your life in time. From either angle, you don't need to grasp anything. You only need to be present.

You need self-verified knowledge, self-understanding, and self-actualization. All of these are like taste. You are the only person on this Earth who can give a taste to yourself.

But don't take this as discouraging news. The whole of Existence supports you in this. The more present you are, the more you experience this support. Everything that exists is supporting you to become who you really are. And at the same time, you have to desire it. You have to wish it.

When you fully participate,
you are fully alive.

To become a unified entity—the direct emanation of your True nature—is a very big aim. At the Breema Center, we refer to that as the Inner Authority, as being present, as taste. But it is one thing really—that which *is*. And what *is*, is always in unity. Reality is always in unity. It has no opposition. Truth includes all opposites within itself.

This is simple. It's beyond thought, feeling, and sensation. It belongs to a dimension that thought, feeling, and sensation can't reach. No amount of thinking can give you insight into the moment. Thinking is a function, but the moment isn't. In the moment, you are *aware* of your thoughts. You know they are not you. They are just thoughts, and they aren't a problem.

Being present means don't live your life in the past and future. Live in the present. Don't go to the past. Bring the past into the present. Instead of imagining yourself back in a past experience, you can remain present while you're looking at the past. This way, you receive useful food from the past. It's the same with the future. Don't go to the future. Prepare yourself by being present now. Now, your Being is participating in your life.

Breema simplifies the process. In everything, it guides us toward building or finding an Inner Authority. The Inner Authority is free from past and future. It is not affected by your mind, feelings, or sensations, and so, can see them objectively, for what they are. Then you see that mind, feelings, and sensations are not you. They are acquired aspects, not you yourself. The more you really see this, the less you identify with your thoughts, feelings, and sensations, and the more you are free to be yourself.

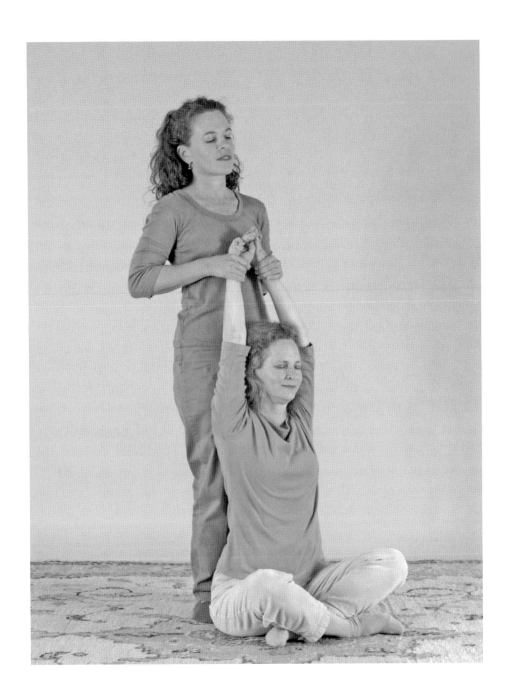

When you come from the past and future to the present, you become available to taste *presence*. This is what happens when you apply the Breema principles. For example, when you try to register body has weight and body breathes, only a small part of the mind is registering. But that little part is free from imaginary past and future. When that grows to the point where the whole mind is registering, that knowing becomes definite—a taste of real knowledge.

When you manifest being present, an echo comes back to you from your activity—*I am present*. It's as simple as that. The Nine Principles are not poetry, not something nice to say, they're the fact of your experience if you are receptive to it. Breema is an activity that supports you to have a momentary experience of being present, and to prolong it a bit, so you can benefit. Once you get what this means, you see it's your birthright to be this way. Why should you be any other way? Why should you be absent?

For so many years, you've lived in your head. What did you get from it? The body breathes—you "know" that, in an automatic way. But now you could know that consciously. You may say, "I don't have time." But you have time to say that sentence, and knowing you are breathing takes less time than that.

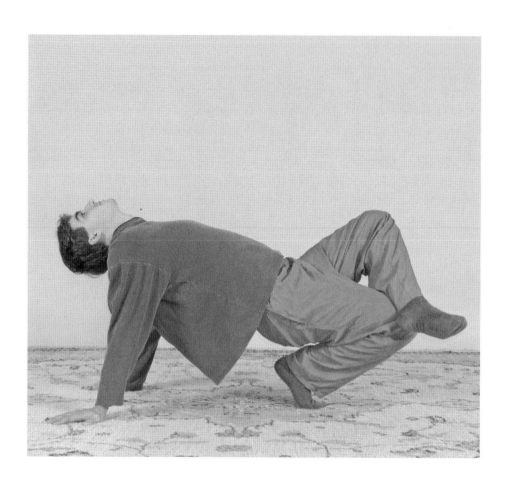

Your Being can't be conditioned. Only your acquired aspect can be conditioned. Mass consciousness has no access to your Being. Your education can't touch it. Your mind can't touch it. Only truth can. That's why you don't have to be worried about your conditioned part, because your Being is untouched.

Breema bodywork reaches your Being by bypassing the mind. Conscious energy is an emanation, and it reaches and nurtures your essence, your Being. The more your essence is nurtured, the less you are subject to your conditioned thoughts, feelings, and movements. When your Being participates in your life, it gives you insights that guide you toward Self-understanding and the ability to manifest in harmony with life.

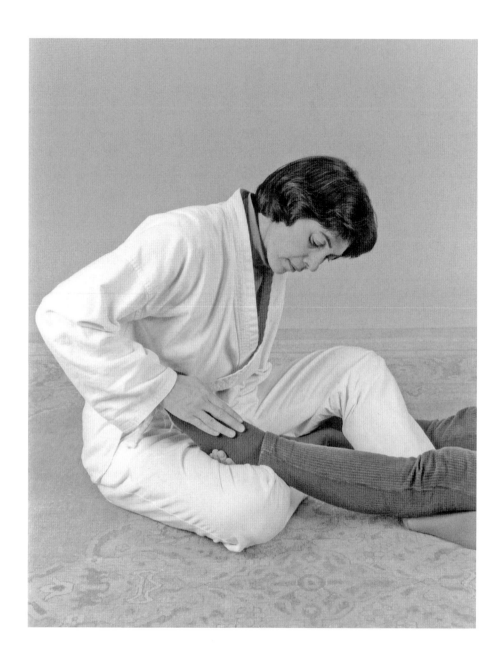

138

What we usually call "doing" refers to an obvious expression of the life force through the activity of the body. But even when the sense organs don't recognize "doing," something is still taking place, because the life force is constantly manifesting. The realizable world has its own activity. We may not recognize it, but that's real doing. So Breema is what we do and what we don't do. Body is moving, but your True nature is also emanating.

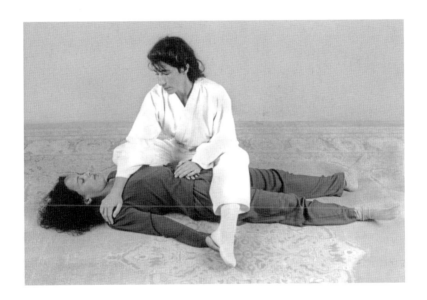

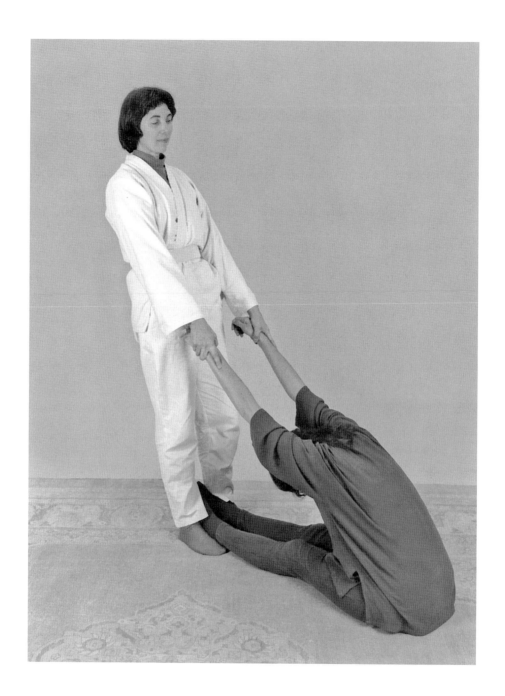

Practicing Breema bodywork offers us the possibility of entering the process of disidentification with ourselves as a name and object, and coming to the unity of body, mind, and feelings. In that unity, we receive Conscious energy. And Conscious energy carries with it all the knowledge in the universe. With it, you can see the essence of things. This is the alchemy that turns lead into gold. Lead is our fragmented, conceptual relationship to life through past and future. Gold is the present moment.

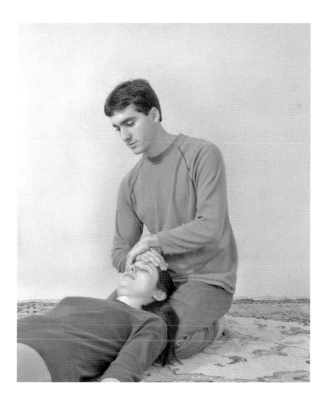

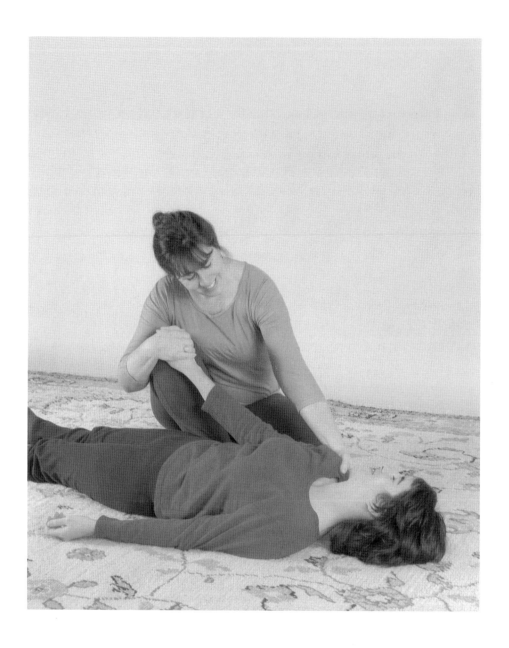

When the mouth expresses what is in the heart, the words aren't extra. Heart is the knowledge of being in unity. Existence expresses itself in the moment, moment by moment. Being wishes to express itself in unity, and it does. It doesn't come out of your past knowledge. When you do Breema, the same principle is manifesting. What your hand communicates is also an expression of the heart, because your receptivity allows Existence to express itself through your touch.

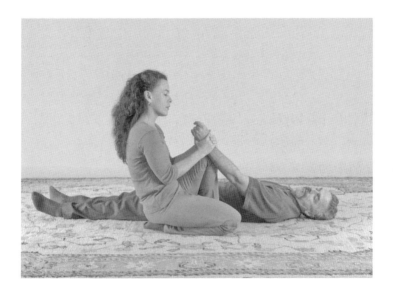

You can't separate Breema bodywork from the philosophy of Breema.

And you can't separate the philosophy of Breema from the philosophy of Existence.

We learn and practice so many Breema sequences, and so many Self-Breema exercises. What is the fruit of it all? The fruit is to come 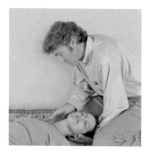 to *taste*. But that's the fruit that's still hanging on the branches, not yet ripe. And unless you eat ripe fruit, you are not fully nurtured by it. How does the fruit ripen? Practicing a lot may be part of it. But what really ripens the fruit is taking taste into your daily life. You may receive tastes while you practice Breema and Self-Breema, and while you are in Breema classes. You have to know that those are tastes of your existence. But then, if you aren't participating in your daily life with that taste, you are not eating ripe fruit.

So we have the Nine Principles. Every one of them can be practiced in your daily life. You don't need to wait until you find someone to practice Breema with, or until you have a chance to do one Self-Breema. If taste becomes a part of you, part of your inner atmosphere, it is with you wherever you are, whatever you do.

Taste is in an entirely differ-ent dimension than the body, thoughts, or feelings. They are all events of life, and together they make up our temporary aspect. But while we have this body, we need to come to know it, to taste it. Taste is the begin-ning of our eternal aspect, which

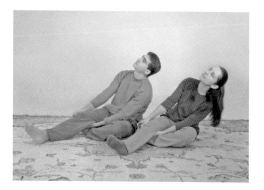

is not dependent on the life of this body. The body, mind, and feelings are born to die. They appear and will disappear. But our reality is Timeless. It is not subject to time, to appearing and disappearing.

The purpose of practicing Breema is to bring us in contact with this eternal aspect. It's to gain true self-knowledge, which can become self-understanding, and eventually self-transformation. The purpose of practicing Breema is to become familiar with taste, and eventually make taste an integral part of your life. Then, instead of living your life mechanically, always moved by outer influences, you could have the dignity of knowing *I exist*. That is the real fruit of Breema.

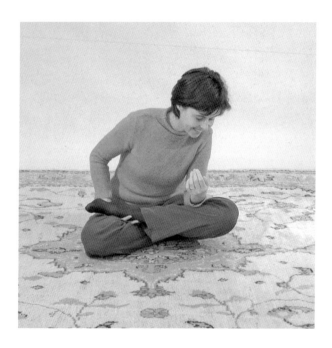

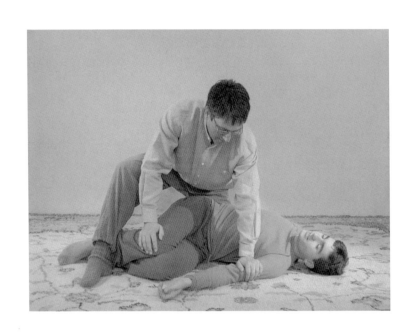

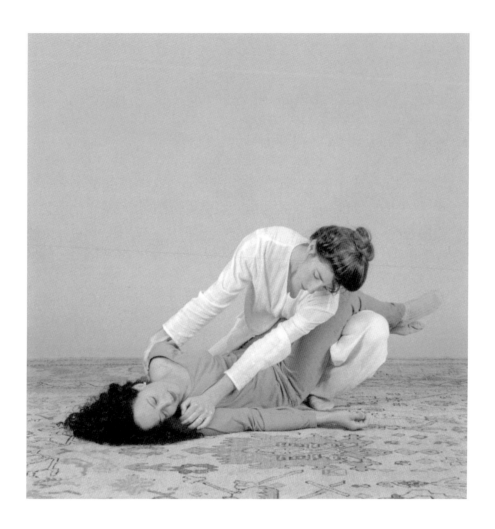

Breema Bodywork

Breema is a unifying, harmonizing method that includes the Nine Principles of Harmony, Breema bodywork, and Self-Breema exercises. Breema bodywork provides an ideal opportunity to actualize the Breema principles. Through practicing and receiving Breema, we can take many steps toward tasting the essential unity of all Existence.

As we practice and deepen our understanding of the principles, Breema gives us a new education in which we learn, first through our body, that the principles are a natural way to relate to ourselves, to other people, and to everything in life.

We can gain a practical understanding of Mutual Support by experiencing that the recipient's body supports our every movement and posture, just as our body simultaneously supports the recipient's.

Through being present and actualizing the principle of No Judgment, an atmosphere of acceptance is created. The experience of touching another body in this nonjudgmental way gives us many glimpses that we are not separate from anything in the universe.

In our ordinary state, we live inside our mind. We practice Breema in order to "come out" of the mind. Breema's principles free us from our mistaken identification with our mind as ourselves. We can let go of the imaginary separation that keeps us from participating fully in life.

The aim of working with the principles of Breema is to come to a level of consciousness in which we know we are not separate from the life that surrounds us, and to see that everything that happens is part of the process of Existence manifesting. In these moments, we are able to conserve the energy we usually waste in judgment and criticism. We have acceptance of whatever we see or experience, based on the recognition of the perfect harmony of life, which dynamically changes form, moment by moment. Seeing that things are the only way they could be in this very moment allows us to use our life energy constructively by fully participating in whatever we are doing.

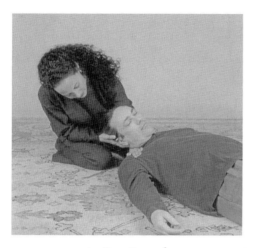

The ability to recognize the nature of life and reality, and to respond harmoniously, are qualities of our Being. Our acquired character never gains this ability. It lacks the strength to get us to do what is right, even if we were to know what that is, because our acquired character is a constantly changing parade of crystallized thoughts and emotions, each of which we assume is "me" at the moment it manifests. These acquired "I's," appearing one after another in time, create our ordinary gross consciousness. We were not responsible for their formation, and in fact, they are not who we really are. They simply represent the functioning of mass consciousness in us, which we mistake for our own consciousness. But our Being is the source of our real consciousness and is conscious of itself as part of Existence. Its authority is real, because its knowledge is real. It has Being-knowledge, which is self-knowledge, inner knowledge. It recognizes reality by tasting reality in itself.

This Being-participation is the aim of Breema bodywork. At the moment our Being participates, we have an Inner Authority that tells us we exist, and this taste of existing is all the support we need to manifest in harmony with Existence. Breema bodywork offers us ideal conditions in which we can take step after step toward becoming

150

present by actualizing the principles inherent in its movements and sequences. Through the support of the atmosphere of acceptance, we can taste many moments of being present.

Eventually, as we gain confidence, we see the opportunity to practice Breema during short moments of other life situations. Our small successes in actualizing a moment, here and there, of being present, encourage us to bring Breema into more of our daily activities. We may even come to the point where we see that nothing is really an obstacle to living our life with the knowledge that *there is a body*, or the knowledge that *I exist* and *Existence exists*. As we enjoy the freedom and harmony of tasting and manifesting our True nature in many situations in life, we become grateful for everything life brings us. Our gratitude becomes a part of the warmth and beauty of life that nurtures us and everyone around us.

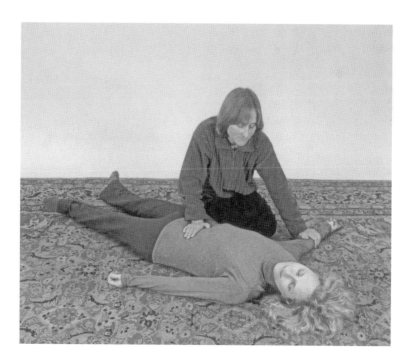

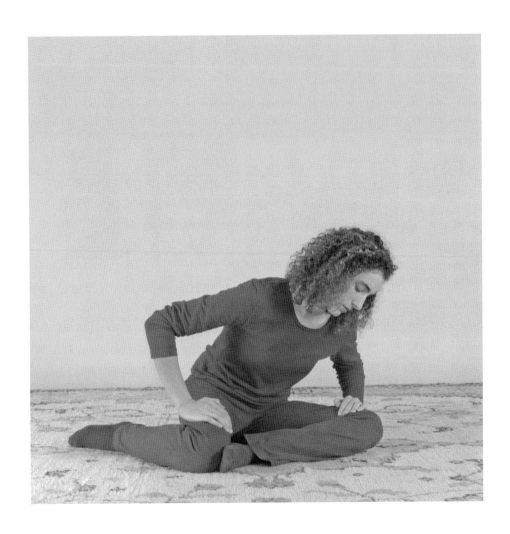

Self-Breema Exercises

Self-Breema exercises are sequences done on one's own body. They are an opportunity to experience being both the practitioner and the recipient at the same time.

The movements of Self-Breema are balanced and in harmony with our essential nature. By working with the Breema principles as we practice Self-Breema, we simplify and purify the activity of the mind and feelings, inviting a higher level of consciousness that is less mechanical and more purposeful to participate in the body's movements.

The physical body is a container. We usually fill it with thoughts and feelings that have a disharmonizing effect on our physiological function. When the container is filled with Consciousness, we experience aliveness and vitality in the body. When Consciousness participates in our activity, the imbalanced vibrations we receive from our surroundings are transformed into harmonious energy that can be beneficially used by the body.

Practicing Self-Breema and the Nine Principles invites physical flexibility, emotional balance, and mental clarity, and helps us to move in harmony with the natural laws that govern life and health. As body, mind, and feelings unite in a common aim, we become present. We experience a natural vitality and a deep connection to all life. As our Being participates in our life, it guides us toward higher levels of consciousness in which we can wake up to our True nature.

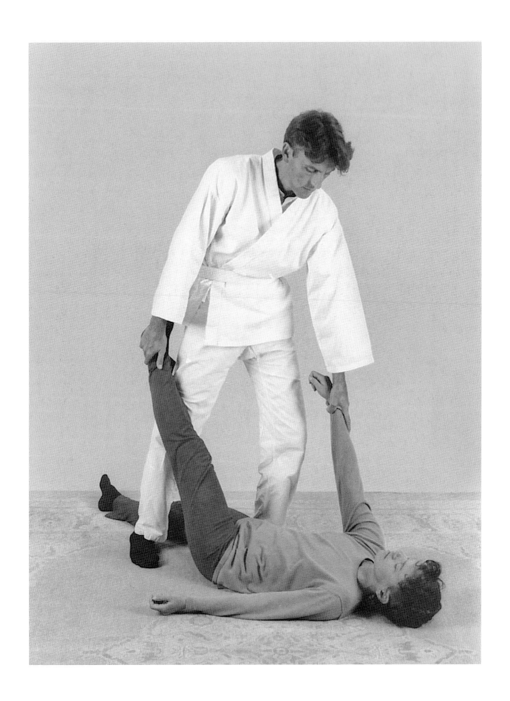

154

The Breema Center

The Breema Center was founded in the early 1980s by myself and a core group of interested colleagues, including: Malouchek Mooshan, Gretchen Brandt, Marian Clark, Janet Madden, J.D. Winitz, Denise Berezonsky, and Roxanne Caswell. We were all interested in a system of health improvement that would not only consider the interrelationships of the body's physiological and structural systems, but would also harmonize the relationship between body, mind, and feelings. I am particularly grateful to Malouchek Mooshan for his contribution of the bodywork and exercises, and for his essential insights into the principles and philosophy of Breema.

Our early classes in Oakland and Berkeley presented a disarmingly simple introduction to the bodywork and principles, and were met with intense interest and enthusiasm. I concurrently opened a clinic, "treating" all my patients with Breema and Self-Breema. The bodywork and exercises created a profound receptivity in patients, and helped them become less subject to rigid, "crystallized" ways of moving, thinking, and feeling.

The next two decades were spent working intensively with a dedicated group of instructors, including all of the original core group. Our aim was to create a diverse yet comprehensive body of sequences and self-exercises that could express the nine universal principles and also serve as an ideal vehicle through which to experience them. We wanted to form Breema and Self-Breema into a system that could illuminate and convey the principles both logically and experientially to the world. The result is Breema bodywork and Self-Breema as they are taught today at the Breema Center.

Over the years, the Breema Center has evolved into a school where the immediate emphasis is on becoming present, unifying body, mind, and feelings, and raising our level of consciousness. Students who come

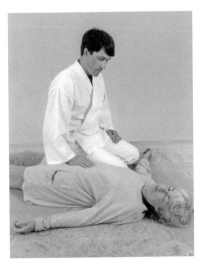

to study Breema bodywork and Self-Breema at the Center quickly discover that Breema's primary importance is not as a bodywork and exercise system. Breema is really for anyone who wants to live a harmonious life by taking a step in the direction of self-verified self-understanding.

I am very grateful that Breema continues to be in the center of my life. I want to always remain a student, and deepen my understanding by working with the principles in all my daily activities. As an instructor, I wish to communicate the essence of Breema in a way that supports students to taste it for themselves. And as the director of the Center, I hope to make Breema accessible to everyone who discovers a sincere interest in it.

If what you read strikes a resonant chord, you really should get a first-hand taste of Breema. Then you can really begin to work with the principles and exercises, and discover the harmonizing effect they can have on your life.

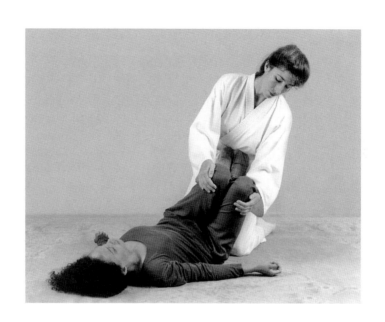

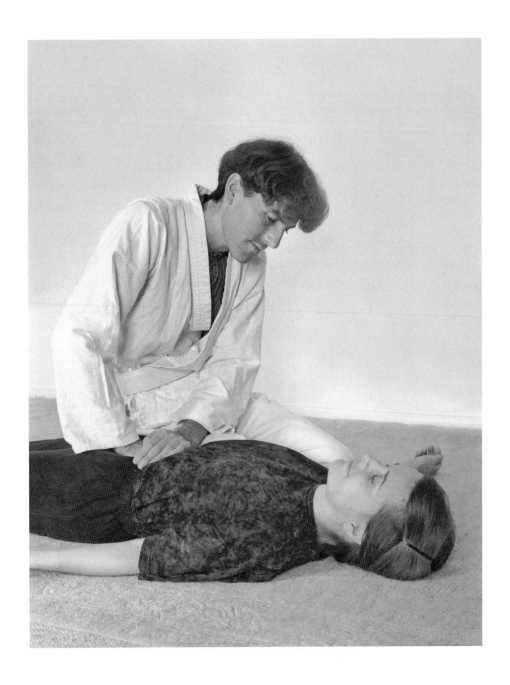

Studying Breema

Since 1980, the Breema Center has been presenting Breema's practical approach to harmony and Self-understanding. The world headquarters for practitioner and instructor certification and continuing education, the Center also gives classes, workshops, and intensives for beginning, intermediate, and advanced students. People come from all over the world, attracted by Breema's philosophy, principles, bodywork, and exercises. Studying at the Center, they find essential support in creating a new, unified relationship between the body, mind, and feelings, and in bringing greater harmony and presence to their lives.

The Breema Center maintains an active relationship with certified practitioners and instructors, and an up-to-date international directory of instructors and practitioners, plus listings of Breema classes and presentations worldwide. Information is available on our website (www. breema.com), or by phone or mail.

THE BREEMA CENTER
Jon Schreiber, D.C., Director
6076 Claremont Avenue
Oakland, CA 94618

510-428-0937
800-452-1008
fax: 510-428-9235

e-mail: center@breema.com
website: www.breema.com

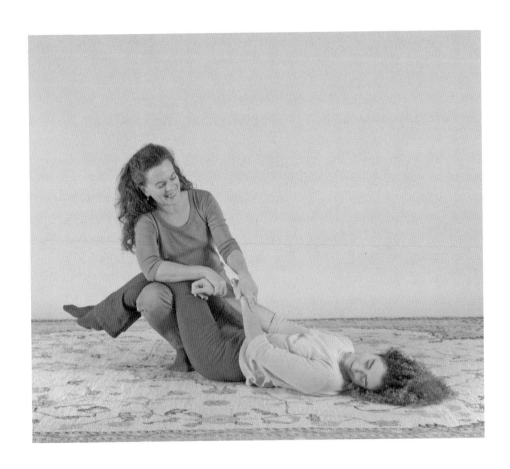

The Breema Clinic

We have been using Breema bodywork, Self-Breema exercises, and working with the principles of Breema since 1981 to help patients find a greater sense of well-being, harmony, and interest in life. Receiving Breema and practicing Self-Breema nurtures our essential interest and helps us move, feel, and think more naturally.

Breema bodywork and Self-Breema exercises are phenomenal catalysts for the body's self-healing processes, and ideal methods of health enhancement for anyone who wishes to benefit from a higher level of physical balance and emotional well-being. They remind us, tangibly yet nonverbally, that real health means harmony with Existence.

THE BREEMA CLINIC
Jon Schreiber, D.C., Director
6201 Florio Street
Oakland, CA 94618

phone: 510-428-1234
fax: 510-428-2705

email: clinic@breema.com
website: www.breemahealth.com

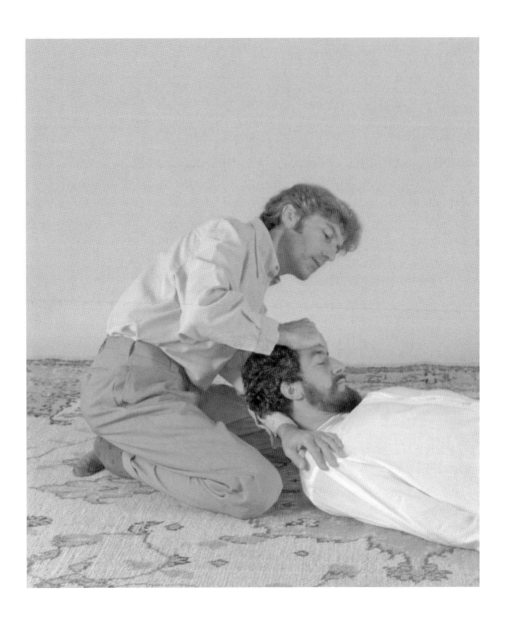

Jon Schreiber

In 1980, Jon Schreiber founded the Breema Center, the world head-quarters for teaching Breema and certifying Breema practitioners and instructors. He is also the founder and director of the Breema Clinic in Oakland, California. He prepared for a traditional medical degree at Columbia University in New York, and subsequently became interested in complementary approaches to health and healing. While completing his Doctor of Chiropractic degree at Palmer College of Chiropractic-West, he began searching for a truly holistic approach to health and life. Working intensively with a group that formed to support this aim, he developed a method that purely expresses the universal principles governing health.

Recognizing the depth and potential of Breema's unique philosophy, principles, method and results, Dr. Schreiber has devoted himself to studying and teaching all aspects of Breema. Besides using Breema and Self-Breema therapeutically to care for patients in his clinic, he maintains an active teaching schedule at the Breema Center, as well as nationally and internationally. Dr. Schreiber is also the author of several books on the philosophy, principles, and practice of Breema bodywork and Self-Breema.

Books from Breema Center Publishing

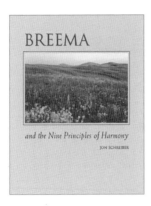

BREEMA *and the* Nine Principles of Harmony

BY JON SCHREIBER

$25.00 hardcover, 168 pages, 7" x 9"
81 photographs

Breema is universal and has great potential value to anyone with a sincere interest in Truth, because it's a practical road to Self-understanding. Breema's timeless principles are applicable to every situation in life, and they open us to the possibility of awakening to the essential unity of Existence in this very moment.

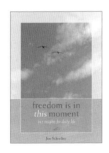

Freedom Is in *This* Moment
365 Insights for Daily Life

BY JON SCHREIBER

$18.95 hardcover, 448 pages, 4½" x 6"

When you read these writings, you are filled up with an inner resonance, because their reality and meaning are in you as well as all around you. When you hear the Truth, you also hear it inside of yourself, in your very essence. The Truth is not something foreign. It's already part of you just because you exist!

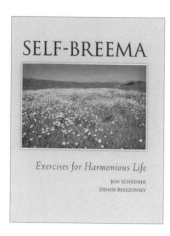

SELF-BREEMA:

Exercises for Harmonious Life

Second Edition

BY JON SCHREIBER &
DENISE BEREZONSKY

$29.95 hardcover, 246 pages, 8½" x 11"
39 photographs, over 400 illustrations

41 fully illustrated Self-Breema exercises and an
introduction to Breema's Nine Principles of Harmony.
Practicing Self-Breema helps us move in unity with
the natural laws that govern life and health, and live in
balance with ourselves, others, and all life.

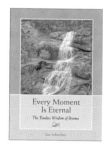

Every Moment Is Eternal

The Timeless Wisdom of Breema

BY JON SCHREIBER

$15.00 hardcover, 200 pages, 4½" x 6"

This book talks to our essential nature, because Truth already exists
there. The more our essence is nurtured, the greater the chance
that cracks may appear in our conditioned attitude towards life.
Through these cracks, we may see things we haven't seen before,
and nourish our essential desire for Self-understanding.

Breema Center Publishing • 6076 Claremont Avenue • Oakland, CA 94618 • U.S.A.
To order books, please call (800) 452-1008
or visit us on the Internet at **www.breema.com**